Diabetes, the Kidney, and Cardiovascular Risk

Guest Editor

GEORGE L. BAKRIS, MD

CARDIOLOGY CLINICS

www.cardiology.theclinics.com

Consulting Editor

MICHAEL H. CRAWFORD, MD

August 2010 • Volume 28 • Number 3

SAUNDERS an imprint of ELSEVIER, Inc.

W.B. SAUNDERS COMPANY
A Division of Elsevier Inc.

1600 John F. Kennedy Blvd. • Suite 1800 • Philadelphia, PA 19103-2899

http://www.theclinics.com

CARDIOLOGY CLINICS Volume 28, Number 3
August 2010 ISSN 0733-8651, ISBN-13: 978-1-4377-2430-1

Editor: Barbara Cohen-Kligerman

Cardiology Clinics (ISSN 0733-8651) is published quarterly by Elsevier Inc., 360 Park Avenue South, New York, NY 10010-1710. Months of issue are February, May, August, and November. Business and Editorial Offices: 1600 John F. Kennedy Blvd., Ste. 1800, Philadelphia, PA 19103-2899. Customer Service Office: 3251 Riverport Lane, Maryland Heights, MO 63043. Periodicals postage paid at New York, NY and additional mailing offices. Subscription prices are $264.00 per year for US individuals, $416.00 per year for US institutions, $132.00 per year for US students and residents, $322.00 per year for Canadian individuals, $517.00 per year for Canadian institutions, $374.00 per year for international individuals, $517.00 per year for international institutions and $187.00 per year for Canadian and international students/residents. To receive student/resident rate, orders must be accompanied by name of affiliated institution, data of term, and the *signature* of program/residency coordinator on institution letterhead. Orders will be billed at individual rate until proof of status is received. Foreign air speed delivery is included in all *Clinics* subscription prices. All prices are subject to change without notice. **POSTMASTER:** Send address changes to *Cardiology Clinics*, Elsevier Health Sciences Division, Subscription Customer Service, 3251 Riverport Lane, Maryland Heights, MO 63043. **Customer Service: 1-800-654-2452 (U.S. and Canada); 314-447-8871 (outside U.S. and Canada). Fax: 314-447-8029. E-mail: journalscustomerservice-usa@elsevier.com (for print support); journalsonlinesupport-usa@elsevier.com (for online support).**

Reprints. For copies of 100 or more, of articles in this publication, please contact the Commercial Reprints Department, Elsevier Inc., 360 Park Avenue South, New York, NY 10010-1710. Tel.: 212-633-3812; Fax: 212-462-1935; E-mail: reprints@elsevier.com.

Cardiology Clinics is also published in Spanish by McGraw-Hill Interamericana Editores S. A., P.O. Box 5-237, 06500, Mexico D. F., Mexico; in Portuguese by Reichmann and Alfonso Editores Rio de Janeiro, Brazil; and in Greek by Dimitrios P. Lagos, 8 Pondon Street, GR115-28 Ilissia, Greece.

Cardiology Clinics is covered in *MEDLINE/PubMed (Index Medicus), Excerpta Medica, The Cumulative Index to Nursing and Allied Health Literature* (CINAHL).

Printed and bound by CPI Group (UK) Ltd, Croydon, CR0 4YY
Transferred to Digital Print 2011

Contributors

CONSULTING EDITOR

MICHAEL H. CRAWFORD, MD
Professor of Medicine and University
of California, San Francisco; Lucie Stern
Chair in Cardiology and Chief of Clinical
Cardiology, University of California,
San Francisco Medical Center,
San Francisco, California

GUEST EDITOR

GEORGE L. BAKRIS, MD, FASN, FASH
Professor of Medicine and Director,
Hypertensive Diseases Unit, The Hypertensive
Diseases Unit/Section of Endocrinology,
Diabetes and Metabolism, The University
of Chicago Pritzker School of Medicine,
Chicago, Illinois

AUTHORS

GEORGE L. BAKRIS, MD, FASN, FASH
Professor of Medicine and Director,
Hypertensive Disease Unit, The Hypertensive
Diseases Unit/Section of Endocrinology,
Diabetes and Metabolism, The University
of Chicago Pritzker School of Medicine,
Chicago, Illinois

DAVID A. CALHOUN, MD
Professor of Medicine, Vascular Biology and
Hypertension Program, University of Alabama
at Birmingham, Birmingham, Alabama

DAN FARBSTEIN, BSc
Candidate for MD-PhD degree, Faculty
of Medicine, Technion-Israel Institute
of Technology, Haifa, Israel

ALLISON J. HAHR, MD
Assistant Professor of Medicine, Division of
Endocrinology, Metabolism, and Molecular
Medicine, Northwestern University Feinberg
School of Medicine, Chicago, Illinois

KEITH A. HOPKINS, MD
Hypertension Fellow, The Hypertensive
Diseases Unit/Section of Endocrinology,
Diabetes and Metabolism, The University
of Chicago Pritzker School of Medicine,
Chicago, Illinois

RIGAS G. KALAITZIDIS, MD, PhD
Senior Registrar in Nephrology, Department
of Nephrology, University Hospital of Ioannina,
Ioannina, Greece

JAY L. KOYNER, MD
Assistant Professor of Medicine, Section
of Nephrology, Department of Medicine,
University of Chicago, Chicago, Illinois

ANDREW P. LEVY, MD, PhD
Associate Professor, Department of Cell
Biology and Anatomy, Faculty of Medicine,
Technion-Israel Institute of Technology,
Haifa, Israel

FRANCESCO LOCATELLI, MD
Professor of Nephrology, Head of
Department of Nephrology, Dialysis and
Renal Transplantation, Alessandro Manzoni
Hospital, Lecco, Italy

MARK E. MOLITCH, MD
Professor of Medicine, Division of
Endocrinology, Metabolism, and Molecular
Medicine, Northwestern University Feinberg
School of Medicine, Chicago, Illinois

TAMAR S. POLONSKY, MD
Fellow, Cardiovascular Prevention and
Epidemiology, Department of Preventive
Medicine, Feinberg School of Medicine,
Northwestern University, Chicago, Illinois

SANDEEP A. SAHA, MD, FACP
Faculty Hospitalist, Providence Sacred Heart
Medical Center; Medical Investigator,
Providence Medical Research Center,
Spokane; Clinical Instructor, Department of
Medicine, University of Washington School of
Medicine, Seattle, Washington

KUMAR SHARMA, MD
Professor of Medicine and Director, Center
for Renal Translational Medicine, University
of California at San Diego/Veterans Affairs
Medical System, La Jolla, California

MATTHEW J. SORRENTINO, MD
Professor, Section of Cardiology,
Department of Medicine, University of
Chicago Pritzker School of Medicine,
Chicago, Illinois

KATHERINE R. TUTTLE, MD, FACP, FASN
Medical and Scientific Director,
Providence Medical Research Center,
Spokane; Clinical Professor, Division of
Nephrology, Department of Medicine,
University of Washington School of
Medicine, Seattle, Washington

SUNEEL M. UDANI, MD, MPH
Nephrology Fellow, Section of Nephrology,
Department of Medicine, University of
Chicago, Chicago, Illinois

**ADAM T. WHALEY-CONNELL, DO, MSPH,
FAHA, FACP, FASN**
Assistant Professor of Medicine,
Division of Nephrology and Hypertension,
Department of Internal Medicine,
Harry S Truman Veterans Affairs Medical
Center, University of Missouri-Columbia
School of Medicine, Columbia, Missouri

Contents

The Contribution of Early Nephropathy to Cardiovascular Risk   427

Tamar S. Polonsky and Francesco Locatelli

Patients with an estimated glomerular filtration rate (eGFR) of less than 60 mL/min per 1.72 m^2, and presence of microalbuminuria (MA), have an increased risk of cardiovascular (CV) events, compared with patients with normal renal function. The strength of the association among patients with a mild reduction in eGFR depends largely on the population studied, whereas the data regarding MA show an elevated risk among both low- and high-risk populations. Patients with mildly reduced eGFR or MA experience a reduction in CV events and progression of renal disease with treatment of CV risk factors. For patients who experience a myocardial infarction, observational data suggest that patients with a mildly reduced eGFR also have improved outcomes with an early invasive strategy, compared with a noninvasive strategy. However, whether targeting therapy to normalize renal function also confers a reduction in CV events remains unknown.

Should Targeting Albuminuria Be Part of a Cardiovascular Risk Reduction Paradigm?   437

Adam T. Whaley-Connell and Rigas G. Kalaitzidis

Cardiovascular disease (CVD) is the leading cause of morbidity and mortality in the United States as well as the rest of the world. Chronic kidney disease (CKD) is considered a CVD risk equivalent. The development of albuminuria has been identified as an additional possible risk marker that is almost unique to patients with CKD and a marker for predicting CVD risk. This review focuses on clinical and epidemiologic evidence regarding the role of albuminuria in the context of CVD development. It reviews the association of albuminuria with other comorbidities associated with increased cardiovascular risk and the modalities aimed at the reduction of albuminuria and maximizing of cardiovascular risk reduction.

Lower Blood Pressure Goals in High-Risk Cardiovascular Patients: Are They Defensible?   447

Keith A. Hopkins and George L. Bakris

This review highlights the paucity of data that support actively decreasing blood pressures (BP) to a level of less than 130/80 mm Hg. Although the data support a lower cardiovascular (CV) event rate with this lower level of pressure in high-risk CV people, early aggressive intervention to prevent levels from going above this mark prevent development of worsening atherosclerosis. Although no trial will ever prove this concept of prevention, common sense and multiple animal experiments support it. Most patients should have their systolic BP reduced to levels well below 140 mm Hg approaching 130 mm Hg, not 140 mm Hg.

The Effects of Heart Failure on Renal Function   453

Suneel M. Udani and Jay L. Koyner

Heart-kidney interactions have been increasingly recognized by clinicians and researchers who study and treat heart failure and kidney disease. A classification system has been developed to categorize the different manifestations of cardiac and renal dysfunction. Work has highlighted the significant negative prognostic effect of worsening renal function on outcomes for individuals with heart failure. The etiology of concomitant cardiac and renal dysfunction remains unclear; however, evidence supports alternatives to the established theory of underfilling, including effects of venous congestion and changes in intra-abdominal pressure. Conventional therapy focuses on blockade of the renin-angiotensin-aldosterone system with expanding use of direct renin and aldosterone antagonists. Novel therapeutic interventions using extracorporeal therapy and antagonists of the adenosine pathway show promise and require further investigation.

Diabetic patients with chronic kidney disease are at high risk for cardiovascular disease (CVD). All aspects of risk reduction should be rigorously applied to such patients. Statins should be used with reduction of low-density lipoprotein cholesterol levels, and blood pressure management is important. Glycemic control remains important for reduction in the development and progression of retinopathy, neuropathy, and even nephropathy itself. Reduction of other risk factors, such as smoking cessation and weight reduction, should also be implemented. Multiple risk factor reduction can have a large effect on reduction of CVD outcomes.

Prospective identification of which individuals with diabetes mellitus (DM) are at greatest risk for developing cardiovascular disease (CVD) complications would have considerable public health importance by allowing the allocation of limited resources to be focused on those individuals who would most benefit from aggressive intervention. Over the past 20 years genetic disease association studies have demonstrated that polymorphisms at specific genetic loci may identify those individuals at greatest risk for developing CVD in the setting of DM. This article reviews the evidence accumulated to date on four polymorphic loci with the aim of explaining how these polymorphisms modify the risk for CVD in DM by modifying the functional activity of a specific gene. Use of the knowledge of these genetic differences among individuals in targeting drug therapy (pharmacogenomics) is also discussed.

Diabetes mellitus leads to the development of a host of micro- and macrovascular complications, which collectively lead to substantial morbidity and mortality. Among the microvascular complications of diabetes, diabetic kidney disease is the most common. Macrovascular complications from diabetes lead to a 2- to 4-fold increase in the incidence of cardiovascular disease and up to twice the mortality from cardiovascular causes as compared with nondiabetic individuals. This article discusses the various drug classes used to treat diabetes mellitus, and reviews the current clinical evidence linking glycemic control using these drug classes on diabetic kidney and cardiovascular disease.

A large body of evidence strongly links aldosterone to development and progression of cardiovascular disease, including vascular stiffness, left ventricular hypertrophy, congestive heart failure, chronic kidney disease, and, especially, hypertension. Emerging data suggest that adipocytes may serve as a source of aldosterone, either directly or indirectly, through the release of aldosterone-stimulating factors. If adipocytes are confirmed to have an important contribution to hyperaldosteronism, it would have significant clinical implications in linking aldosterone to obesity-related increases in cardiovascular risk. Such a cause-and-effect situation would then provide the opportunity to reverse that risk with preferential use of aldosterone antagonists in obese patients.

Early Intervention Strategies to Lower Cardiovascular Risk in Early Nephropathy: Focus on Dyslipidemia   529

Matthew J. Sorrentino

Patients with chronic kidney disease (CKD) are at high cardiovascular risk and we can consider them to have a risk equivalent to coronary heart disease, putting them into the high-risk category. A mixed dyslipidemia with high triglyceride levels; low high-density lipoprotein (HDL) levels; and small, dense low-density lipoprotein (LDL) particles is a common pattern in patients with CKD, contributing to their high cardiovascular disease (CVD) risk. A treatment strategy to reduce LDL cholesterol to the current high-risk category goals reduces risk similar to patients without CKD. Emerging evidence suggests that targeting non-HDL cholesterol can have the potential to bring about further CVD risk reduction. Non-HDL cholesterol should be a secondary target for all patients with CKD. Further studies are needed to determine the magnitude of the risk reduction we can expect to gain by targeting non-HDL cholesterol and the most effective way to treat this target.

Cardiology Clinics

VISIT OUR WEB SITE!
Access your subscription at:
www.theclinics.com

Foreword

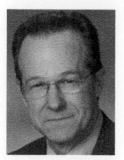

Michael H. Crawford, MD
Consulting Editor

Chronic kidney disease is a known risk factor for, or cotraveler with, cardiovascular disease. Chronic kidney disease patients often have traditional atherosclerotic risk factors, such as hypertension, dyslipidemia, and diabetes. In addition, they may have unique endothelial dysfunction often manifested as albuminuria. Also, the combination of renal dysfunction and cardiovascular disease often leads to a vicious cycle of rapid deterioration in renal and cardiac function. Finally, there is the problem that treatment of cardiovascular disease may worsen renal disease and vice versa. A classic example is the diminution in renal function when very high blood pressures in chronic kidney disease patients are quickly returned to normal pharmacologically.

This issue of *Cardiology Clinics* addresses these issues and more. George Bakris, the Guest Editor, is one of the foremost authorities on cardiorenal function and has assembled an outstanding group of experts to discuss this topic. It is noteworthy that he chose a nephrologist and a cardiologist to discuss each topic. Many practical patient care issues are addressed, such as the effect of heart failure on renal function, how low blood pressure should be lowered in patients with chronic kidney disease, and what should be done about albuminuria. As the percentage of the population that is elderly increases, these issues will become more prevalent, and optimal care of patients with renal and cardiovascular disease will depend on knowledge about the issues discussed in this issue.

Michael H. Crawford, MD
Division of Cardiology
Department of Medicine
University of California
San Francisco Medical Center
505 Parnassus Avenue, Box 0124
San Francisco, CA 94143-0124, USA

E-mail address:
crawfordm@medicine.ucsf.edu

doi:10.1016/j.ccl.2010.05.001

cardiology.theclinics.com

Preface

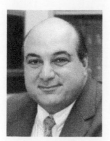

George L. Bakris, MD
Guest Editor

The importance of kidney dysfunction in the context of cardiovascular risk is now well validated. Those with an estimated glomerular filtration rate below 45 mL/min are known to have more than a 3-fold higher risk of myocardial infarction and stroke as well as a higher risk of heart failure. The mechanisms that portend this higher cardiovascular risk are not well delineated, but more recent studies are helping to elucidate the role of various markers, such as microalbuminuria, in understanding the contribution of kidney dysfunction to endothelial dysfunction. The articles in this issue were coauthored, for the most part, by nephrologists and cardiologists so that the approaches and attitudes of each discipline could be captured. We hope that these new insights into the common problem of kidney disease contributing to heart disease expands readers' knowledge and breadth of approach to aid in better management of patients.

George L. Bakris, MD
The Hypertensive Diseases Unit
Section of Endocrinology
Diabetes and Metabolism
The University of Chicago
Pritzker School of Medicine
5841 South Maryland Avenue, MC 1027
Chicago, IL 60637, USA

E-mail address:
gbakris@gmail.com

Cardiol Clin 28 (2010) xi
doi:10.1016/j.ccl.2010.04.010
0733-8651/10/$ – see front matter © 2010 Elsevier Inc. All rights reserved.

The Contribution of Early Nephropathy to Cardiovascular Risk

Tamar S. Polonsky, MD[a], Francesco Locatelli, MD[b],*

KEYWORDS

- Glomerular filtration rate • Microalbuminuria
- Cardiovascular disease

It is well established that the presence of chronic kidney disease (CKD) is associated with a significant increase in the risk of cardiovascular disease (CVD).[1] Patients with CKD are far more likely to develop CVD than they are to develop end-stage renal disease.[2] However, whether patients with only mild kidney disease, as measured by glomerular filtration rate, are also at greater risk for cardiovascular events is less clear. On the other hand, the presence of microalbuminuria (MA) is also categorized as mild kidney disease, and substantial data suggest that patients with MA experience a higher cardiovascular (CV) event rate than those without MA, even at levels below the threshold for the diagnosis of MA.

This article discusses some data regarding how the presence of a mildly reduced glomerular filtration rate or MA affects cardiovascular risk. It also explores some of the potential explanations of the findings and evaluates the effect of medical therapy on cardiovascular risk and progression of renal dysfunction.

DEFINITION OF MILDLY IMPAIRED RENAL FUNCTION

Patients may be diagnosed with mild nephropathy based on the presence of either mildly reduced estimated glomerular filtration rate (eGFR), which represents overall kidney function; or the presence of MA, which represents damage specifically to the glomerulus. The current preferred method to derive the eGFR is the Modification of Diet in Renal Disease study equation:[3]

$$186 \times SCr^{-1.154} \times Age^{-0.203} \times (0.742 \text{ if female}) \times (1.210 \text{ if black})$$

where SCr is serum creatinine concentration in milligrams per deciliter; age is in years, and weight is in kilograms.

A normal eGFR is greater than 90 mL/min/1.73 m^2 of body surface area, and a mild reduction in eGFR is 60 to 89 mL/min/1.73 m^2. Estimated GFR is the preferred index to establish baseline kidney function, because it is more sensitive than creatinine.[3] Substantial reductions in eGFR may exist in the setting of a normal creatinine. For example, depending on a person's age, gender, and race, an eGFR of 60 could correspond to a creatinine of 0.95 to 1.73 mg/dL. Earlier studies looking at the relationship between renal function and cardiovascular outcomes relied on creatinine; in this article, only studies using eGFR will be mentioned.

MA, which refers to albumin excretion that exceeds the normal range but is below the minimum level for detection by tests for total protein, is defined as 30 to 299 mg/g on a spot urine albumin–creatinine ratio.[3] Patients with stage 1 kidney disease have a normal eGFR with MA, and patients with stage 2 kidney disease

[a] Cardiovascular Prevention and Epidemiology, Department of Preventive Medicine, Feinberg School of Medicine, Northwestern University, 680 North Lakeshore Drive, Suite 1400, Chicago, IL 60611, USA
[b] Department of Nephrology, Dialysis and Renal Transplantation, Alessandro.Manzoni Hospital, Via Dell'Eremo 9, IT 23900, Lecco, Italy
* Corresponding author.
E-mail address: f.locatelli@ospedale.lecco.it

Cardiol Clin 28 (2010) 427–436
doi:10.1016/j.ccl.2010.04.007

have an eGFR 60 to 89 mL/min/1.73 m^2 with or without MA. Although a 24-hour urine collection may provide important information regarding electrolyte and protein intake, using a sample from the first void in the morning has been shown to be accurate for the diagnosis of MA.[3]

ASSOCIATION OF MILDLY REDUCED EGFR WITH CVD

The prevalence of mildly reduced renal function depends on the population being studied. In the National Health and Nutrition Examination Surveys (NHANES) 1999 to 2000, which include a representative sample of men and women in the United States aged 20 to 75 years, approximately 36% of the population had an eGFR of 60 to

89 mL/min/1.73 m^2; this is in contrast to the Atherosclerosis Risk in the Communities (ARIC) study, an observational study of men and women aged 45 to 64 years, in which almost 50% of the population had mildly reduced kidney function.[2,4]

Several epidemiologic studies have examined whether patients with a mildly reduced eGFR have an increased risk of CVD (**Table 1**). However, the studies' results again vary based on the population being studied. NHANES III compared participants within each category of eGFR, and showed a clear association between the severity of renal dysfunction and cardiovascular risk factors after adjustment for age. For example, 3.4% of participants with an eGFR greater than 90 mL/min/1.73 m^2 have diabetes, compared with 6.2% of those with an eGFR of

Table 1
Summary of selected studies that examined the association of mildly reduced estimated glomerular filtration rate and cardiovascular events

Study	Patient Characteristics	Primary Endpoint	Risk of a Cardiovascular Event, Compared to Individuals with Normal Renal Function
NHANES 1999–2000[2]	Men and women ages 20–75 Mean age 53 6.2% diabetes 26% hypertension	Cardiovascular disease mortality	Adjusted RR 1.48 (95% CI 1.13–1.93)
ARIC[4]	Men and women ages 45–64 Mean age 55 9.6% diabetes 33.6% hypertension 5.5% known CHD	Atherosclerotic cardiovascular disease (MI, cardiac procedure, CHD death, stroke)	Event rate of 6.6%, compared with 5.5% among participants with normal renal function Every 10 mL/min/1.73 m^2 decrease corresponded to a 5%–6% increase in events
Rotterdam Study[5]	Men and women over age 55 Mean age 70 Mean SBP 139.6 mm Hg 10% diabetes	MI	Adjusted HR 1.34 (95% CI 0.89–2.01) among quartile with mean eGFR 78 mL/min/1.73 m^2 Adjusted HR 1.66 (95% CI 1.14–2.49) among quartile with mean eGFR 70 mL/min/1.73 m^2
WHS[6]	Women age ≥45 years Mean age 55–56 24%–25% hypertension 2% diabetes	Nonfatal MI, nonfatal stroke, coronary revascularization, cardiovascular death	Adjusted HR 0.86 (95% CI 0.73 to 1.03) for mean eGFR 60–74 mL/min/1.73 m^2 Adjusted HR 0.93 (0.81 to 1.06) for mean eGFR 75–89 mL/min/1.73 m^2

Abbreviations: ARIC, Atherosclerosis Risk in Communities; CHD, coronary heart disease; CI, confidence interval; HR, hazard ratio; MI, myocardial infarction; NHANES, National Health and Nutrition examination Surveys; RR, relative risk; WHS, Women's Health Study.

60 to 89 mL/min/1.73 m^2, and 15.8% of those with an eGFR 15 to 59 mL/min/1.73 m^2 (P<.001).[2] Mean low-density lipoprotein cholesterol level in individuals with an eGFR 60 to 89 mL/min/1.73 m^2 was 131.6 mg/dL, compared with 118.4 and 144.1 mg/dL for participants with an eGFR of greater than 90 mL/min/1.73 m^2 and 15 to 59 mL/min/1.73 m^2 respectively (P = .003). Persons with an eGFR 60 to 89 experienced a modest increase in CVD mortality with a relative risk (RR) of 1.48 (95% confidence interval [CI] 1.13 to 1.93) after controlling for traditional CV risk factors, but did not have an increase in all-cause mortality. Data from the ARIC study also showed a small increase in the risk of CV events. Individuals with an eGFR 60 to 89 mL/min/1.73 m^2 had an event rate of 6.6%, compared with 5.5% for those with normal renal function, and 14.2% for those with CKD.[4] When eGFR was treated as a continuous variable, a 10 mL/min/1.73 m^2 decrease corresponded to a 5% to 6% increase in the risk of de novo or recurrent events. In addition, the Rotterdam Study, a prospective population-based cohort study of men and women over age 55 years divided participants into quartiles, based on their eGFR.[5] Participants in the second, third, and fourth quartiles had mean eGFRs of 70, 78 and 94 mL/min/1.73 m^2 respectively. After adjusting for CV risk factors, the hazard ratio (HR) for incident myocardial infarction (MI) was 1.34 (95% CI 0.89 to 2.01) in the third quartile and 1.66 (95% CI, 1.14 to 2.49) among participants in the second quartile, compared with participants with normal renal function.

In contrast, in the Women's Health Study, which included a relatively healthy population of women without known CVD, mildly impaired renal function was not associated with an increased risk of CV events.[6] The conflicting results between WHS and the other studies likely reflect the minor role that a mild reduction in eGFR plays in CV risk, making its significance more susceptible to the population in which it is studied. The overall event rate in WHS was lower than in NHANES and ARIC, and the participants had a lower cardiovascular risk factor burden. As a result, it may be that in a younger healthy population the presence of mild renal impairment does not significantly contribute to CV risk. When mild renal impairment is found in the setting of additional CV risk factors, however, it contributes a modest amount to the risk of CV events.

There are several potential explanations why a mild reduction in eGFR would increase the risk of developing CVD. First, there may be residual confounding from traditional CV risk factors, even after adjustment. A decreased eGFR may simply represent vascular damage from a longer duration of risk factors or inadequate control. Second, a decrease in the level of kidney function may result in the accumulation of nontraditional risk factors, such as remnant cholesterol particles or homocysteine, which are not routinely measured.[4] Third, reduced kidney function may lead to structural changes in both central and peripheral arteries. For example, in an observational study of 305 patients with essential hypertension who were free of CVD, those with an eGFR less than 106 mL/min/1.73 m^2 had increased aortic stiffness, compared with those with an eGFR greater than 117 mL/min/1.73 m^2.[7]

Data regarding the clinical outcomes of individuals with a mildly reduced eGFR who experience an MI mirror the data for their risk of a de novo event; those who have mildly reduced renal function have a slightly higher risk for mortality after MI. Using a nationally representative sample of more than 100,000 Medicare patients hospitalized with an acute MI, Smith and colleagues[8] found that, after adjusting for comorbidities and hospital events, patients with an eGFR of 66 to 74 mL/min/1.73 m^2 experienced a 12% higher 1-year mortality, and a 5% higher 10-year mortality, compared with those with normal renal function. Results from the Valsartan in Acute Myocardial Infarction Trial (VALIANT) highlighted the influence of mildly reduced renal function among high-risk patients, even when they received treatment that inhibits the renin–angiotensin system.[9] In the trial, patients who experienced an acute MI that was complicated by either clinical signs of heart failure or systolic dysfunction were randomized to valsartan, captopril, or both. After adjustment for treatment received and comorbidities, patients with an eGFR 60 to 74 mL/min/1.73 m^2 had an adjusted HR of 1.14 for cardiovascular death (95% CI 1.02 to 1.27), and 1.10 for a combined endpoint of CV death, reinfarction, congestive heart failure, and stroke (95% CI, 1.02 to 1.19).

An additional factor that may contribute to the increase in morbidity and mortality of patients with mild renal dysfunction is that they are sometimes treated less intensively than patients with normal renal function. For example, in VALIANT, patients with mildly reduced renal function were slightly less likely to receive therapies such as coronary catheterization (27.5% vs 34.7%), and beta-blockers (71.9% vs 74.7%) compared with patients with normal renal function.[9] The reasons for this are unclear, but could reflect a concern among physicians that patients with mildly reduced renal function would experience more adverse effects or were at higher risk for complications during procedures.

TREATMENT OF CARDIOVASCULAR RISK FACTORS AND EVENTS

Given that patients with mild renal dysfunction are potentially at increased risk both for experiencing a CV event and for complications afterward, it is important to determine whether particular treatment strategies are more effective than others. National Kidney Foundation (NKF) guidelines recommend that treatment of comorbid conditions such as hypertension, interventions to slow progression of kidney disease, and measures to reduce the risk for CVD should begin during stage 1 and stage 2.[3] For example, more than 80% of patients with stage 2 nephropathy have hypertension.[10] Exactly how NKF recommendations should be followed, however, is not well-established. There are no randomized clinical trials focused on patients with early kidney disease to determine the ideal strategy for risk factor modification.

Available data are limited to post-hoc analyses of a few large clinical trials that stratified participants by eGFR. An additional limitation is that most trials analyzed participants with normal and mild renal dysfunction together, although some trials separated the two groups. For example, unadjusted data from the Antihypertensive and Lipid-Lowering Treatment to Prevent Heart Attack Trial (ALLHAT) trial suggest that chlorthalidone may be more effective than amlodipine at reducing heart failure, and marginally more effective than lisinopril at reducing combined CVD events.[11] The data were not adjusted for baseline characteristics, however, significantly limiting the ability to draw firm conclusions. ALLHAT enrolled patients with hypertension and at least one additional risk factor for CHD, whereas two additional trials— Prevention of Events with ACE Inhibition (PEACE) and European Trial on the Reduction of Cardiac Events with Perindopril (EUROPA)—compared the use of an ACEI or placebo specifically in patients with known stable CHD.[12,13] Participants in the ACEI group in both studies achieved a mean systolic blood pressure of about 128 mm Hg, and yet the treatment results in relation to renal function were different. PEACE showed that only participants with an eGFR <60 mL/min/1.73 m^2 derived added benefit from ACEI therapy. EUROPA showed that patients at all levels of renal function experienced a reduction in cardiovascular death, MI, or resuscitated cardiac arrest if they were randomized to ACEI therapy (HR 0.82, 95% CI 0.72 to 0.93, for patients with an eGFR <90

mL/min/1.73 m^2). The authors pointed to the greater proportion of patients achieving the target dose and longer follow-up in the EUROPA trial as potential explanations for the disparate results.[12] Given that the participants in both trials achieved similar blood pressure reduction, it may be that the higher doses of ACE inhibition achieved in EUROPA provided benefits beyond blood pressure lowering, such as direct effects on oxidative stress or endothelial function.

Two lipid-lowering trials suggest that use of statins is not only safe in patients with mild renal dysfunction, but also may attenuate further loss of kidney function. Although in both studies investigators did not distinguish between normal or mildly reduced eGFR. Most participants in the Scandinavian Simvastatin Survival Study (4S), which enrolled more than 4000 men and women with CHD and hyperlipidemia, had an eGFR greater than 60 when the study began.[14] Those randomized to simvastatin 20 mg were almost one third less likely to experience a loss of kidney function that was greater than 25%, compared with participants taking placebo. Results from the Treating to New Targets (TNT) study, which randomized 10,000 men and women with stable CHD to either 10 mg or 80 mg of atorvastatin, suggested that the renoprotective effect of statins may be dose-dependent.[15] Mean eGFR increased in both treatment groups, with a mean change from baseline of 3.5 mL/min per 1.73 m^2 with 10 mg of atorvastatin and 5.2 mL/min per 1.73 m^2 with 80 mg of atorvastatin. Among participants with a baseline eGFR greater than or equal to 60 mL/min per 1.73 m^2, significantly fewer in the 80 mg group declined to less than 60 mL/min per 1.73 m^2 at the end of the study than in the 10 mg group (6.6 vs 9.2%; $P<.0001$).

Both clinical trials and registry studies have attempted to address the effect of mild renal dysfunction among patients treated with percutaneous coronary intervention (PCI). Patients with mild renal dysfunction had slightly lower rates of PCI compared with patients with normal renal function (46% vs 53%) in a Swedish registry, which may partly explain why they are found to have a higher mortality rate.[16] However, for those undergoing angiography, patients with mild renal dysfunction were shown to have similar rates of one-, two-, and three-vessel disease as patients with normal renal function. Further, those with mild renal impairment experienced a 25% to 35% reduction in 6-month and 1-year mortality, with an early invasive strategy for the management of acute coronary syndrome (ACS).[16] Patients with mild renal impairment from a Canadian registry experienced a slight increase in minor bleeding with an invasive strategy compared with patients with normal renal function (0.9% vs 0.4%) and access site complications (1.8% vs 0.6%).[17] None of the studies reported whether patients with mild renal dysfunction were at increased risk of contrast nephropathy.

ASSOCIATION OF MICROALBUMINURIA WITH CVD

MA is thought to occur because of increased leakage of albumin through the capillary wall in the glomerulus, resulting from increased intraglomerular pressure or permeability.[18] Both hypertension and diabetes are the primary risk factors for MA, and both have been shown to increase pressure in the glomerulus; hyperglycemia also has been shown to alter what proteins the glomerulus is able to filter based on positive or negative charge.[18]

As with reduced eGFR, the prevalence of MA varies substantially with the population studied. Data from NHANES showed that 7.4% of the general population has MA, compared with 1.1% with macroalbuminuria.[2] In the Framingham Offspring cohort, in which most participants were ages 50 to 70, the prevalence of MA was 12.2%.[19] However, MA is found primarily in patients with hypertension or diabetes. It is estimated that MA is found in up to 37% of patients with hypertension, and up to 43% of patients with diabetes.[20] Additional risk factors associated with the development of MA are tobacco use, low high-density cholesterol, and abdominal obesity.[21]

The presence of MA signifies ongoing vascular damage, and is associated with several cardiac abnormalities. In the Losartan Intervention for Endpoint Reduction (LIFE) trial, in which patients with stages 1 to 3 hypertension were randomized to losartan or atenolol, more than twice as many participants with MA were found to have concentric hypertrophy in the echocardiography substudy, compared with those with normal renal function (29.6% vs 13.5%, P<.001).[22] A population-based observational study of men and women also showed that MA is associated with cardiac abnormalities. Participants in the Strong Heart Study with MA were more likely to have abnormal diastolic filling.[23] In a study of 308 patients undergoing elective coronary angiography, there was a stepwise increase in the degree of MA as the number of diseased vessels increased.[24]

The relationship between MA and the risk of future CV events has been shown consistently, both in populations with and without traditional CV risk factors (**Table 2**).[19,25,26] In the Heart

Outcomes Prevention Evaluation (HOPE) study, which enrolled participants with known CVD or diabetes, participants with baseline MA experienced a 1.83-fold higher risk of MI, stroke, or CV death (95% CI 1.64 to 2.05) and congestive heart failure hospitalization by 3.23-fold (95% CI, 2.54 to 4.10).[26] In a Danish cohort of individuals with borderline hypertension, the risk of ischemic heart disease increased fourfold in the presence of MA.[27] Importantly, many studies have shown that the risk for CV events that is associated with MA exists in a continuous manner. Even patients well below the cutoff for MA experience an elevated risk for events, and there is no clear plateau as the degree of MA rises.[26,28–30]

The precise mechanism linking MA with CVD is not clear; however, it appears that MA is associated with endothelial dysfunction and inflammation, well-established precursors to the development of atherosclerosis.[18] For example, in the Copenhagen City Heart Study, healthy participants with elevated urinary albumin excretion, many of whom were below the threshold for MA, had decreased flow-mediated dilation, compared with participants with no urinary albumin excretion.[31] In a study that compared patients with hypertension and normal controls, plasma levels of vascular cell adhesion molecule (VCAM) and intracellular adhesion molecule (ICAM), which are markers of endothelial activation, were the highest in those with hypertension and MA.[32] Further, in 328 patients with diabetes followed over 9 years, levels of plasma von-Willebrand factor, soluble E-selectin, and tissue-type plasminogen activator; additional markers of endothelial activation; and C-reactive protein, a marker of inflammation, all independently predicted the development of urinary albumin excretion over time.[33] Some authors, however, have suggested that the link between MA and CVD cannot be fully explained by its association with inflammation and endothelial dysfunction.[34] After adjusting for the levels of circulating biomarkers, MA is still an independent predictor of CVD mortality, suggesting that additional pathways are involved but have not yet been described. It is possible that the presence of MA also fosters a prothrombotic state, or that the presence of MA creates a susceptibility to further vascular damage.[34,35]

TREATMENT OF PATIENTS WITH MICROALBUMINURIA

Given the clear association of MA with CV risk, the diagnosis of MA could identify patients who would

Table 2
Summary of selected studies that examined the association of microalbuminuria and cardiovascular events

Study	Patient Characteristics	Primary Endpoint	Risk of a Cardiovascular Event, Compared with Individuals with Normal Renal Function
NHANES 1999–2002[2]	Men and women ages 20–75 Mean age 39 if including only participants with eGFR >90 mL/min/1.73 m^2 3.4% diabetes 12% hypertension	CV disease mortality	Adjusted RR 2.18 (95% CI 1.45–3.20)
HOPE[26]	Men and women age ≥55 with known Cardiovascular disease or diabetes and one additional risk factor	MI, stroke, CV death, or CHF	Adjusted RR for MI, stroke or CV death 1.83 (95% CI 1.64–2.05) Adjusted RR for CHF 3.23 (95% CI 2.54–4.1)
Framingham Offspring Study[30]	Men and women free of CV disease, hypertension, and diabetes 98/1568 (6%) participants had MA	MI, CHD death, stroke, CHF	Participants with level of MA above the median experienced HR 4.26; 95% CI, 1.70 to 10.66
MONICA[27]	Men and women ages 30–60 free from Ischemic heart disease and diabetes 10% Hypertension	Fatal or nonfatal MI, angina pectoris	Adjusted RR 3.5 (95% CI 1.0 to 12.1)

Abbreviations: CHD, coronary heart disease; CHF, congestive heart failure; CV, cardiovascular; HOPE, Heart Outcomes Prevention Evaluation; HR, hazard ratio; MI, myocardial infarction; MONICA, Monitoring of Trends and Determinants in Cardiovascular Disease; NHANES, National Health and Nutrition Examination Surveys; RR, relative risk.

benefit from aggressive management of CV risk factors. It is therefore recommended that patients at risk for MA, including those with hypertension, diabetes, metabolic syndrome, tobacco use, and age over 60 years undergo screening with a morning void urine albumin–creatinine ratio.[3]

Antihypertensive therapy is a mainstay of treatment for patients with MA. Current guidelines recommend a goal blood pressure of less than 140/90 for the general population, and less than 130/80 for patients with diabetes, although patients who are normotensive have demonstrated reductions from use of blockers of the renin angiotensin system. The greatest amount of clinical trial evidence supports the use of ACEI and angiotensin receptor blockers, both to reduce the progression

to overt nephropathy and decrease CV risk.[20,36] In a cohort of diabetic patients with MA but without hypertension, treatment with enalapril 10 mg stabilized their MA over a mean follow-up of 7 years.[37] In the HOPE trial, in which 31% of the population had MA, treatment with ramipril 10 mg reduced the risk of the combined endpoint of CV death, MI, or stroke by more than 20%, compared with placebo, and reduced the progression to overt nephropathy.[28] Use of losartan in the LIFE trial led to a 33% reduction in the albumin–creatinine ratio at years 1 and 2, compared with a 15% reduction on atenolol.[38] Patients in the highest quartile of albumin excretion achieved the largest reduction in CV events with losartan, although this included patients with macroalbuminuria as well. A prespecified secondary analysis evaluated how changes in MA affected CV risk while receiving treatment. For patients whose baseline MA level was above the median, but then decreased to below the median while receiving therapy, risk of a CV event decreased, compared with participants whose level of MA either stayed the same or increased. This suggests that tracking the level of MA over time may be helpful to gauge the adequacy of treatment.

Although ACEI and angiotensin 2 receptor antagonists (ARB) therapy have been shown individually to improve outcomes in patients with MA, results from the Ongoing Telmisartan Alone and in Combination with Ramipril Global Endpoint Trial (ONTARGET) suggest no added benefit from combining the two drug classes.[36,39] Despite a greater reduction in blood pressure among participants randomized to ramipril plus telmisartan than among participants receiving ramipril or telmisartan monotherapy, the CV event rate was similar between the three groups. In contrast, the rates of discontinuation for hypotensive symptoms, syncope, diarrhea, and renal dysfunction were significantly higher in the participants receiving dual therapy. There was also no additional reduction in CV events seen with combination therapy over monotherapy among the 13% of the study population with MA at baseline, despite a modest decrease in the progression to macroalbuminuria.

Beta-blocker therapy is a potential second-line choice for patients who are not yet at their blood pressure goal. Cardioselective beta-blockers, such as metoprolol and atenolol have been shown to have modest effects on progression of renal disease, and they are the cornerstone of therapy for CHD.[20] However, results from the Glycemic Effects in Diabetes Mellitus Carvedilol-Metoprolol Comparison in Hypertensives (GEMINI) trial suggest that carvedilol may be a more effective medication for patients with MA.[40] Patients with diabetes were all treated with either an ACEI or ARB, and then randomized to carvedilol, (a beta-blocker that also has alpha-blocking properties), or metoprolol. After 5 months of therapy, blood pressure reduction was comparable, but the carvedilol group achieved a 16.2% greater reduction in microalbuminuria than the metoprolol group. The authors proposed that known antioxidant effects seen with carvedilol may reduce vascular injury, and therefore have a beneficial effect on renal function.

Combination therapy with an ACEI and amlodipine is another treatment option, based on results from the Avoiding Cardiovascular Events through Combination Therapy in Patients Living with Systolic Hypertension (ACCOMPLISH) trial.[41] Patients with hypertension and at least one other risk factor for CVD were randomized to a fixed combination of the ACEI benazepril and the dihydropyridine calcium channel blocker amlodipine or benazepril and the diuretic hydrochlorothiazide. Most of the study population had an eGFR greater than 60 mL/min per 1.73 m^2. The trial was stopped early because of a 20% reduction in cardiovascular risk seen in the patients receiving benazepril and amlodipine. In a prespecified analysis, participants randomized to benazepril and amlodipine had a slower decline in eGFR after 2.9 years (−0.88 mL/min/1.73 m^2) compared with those receiving benazepril and hydrochlorothiazide (−4.22 mL/min/1.73 m^2, $P = .01$).[42] Among those receiving benazepril and amlodipine, there was also an almost 50% reduction in the number of participants who experienced a doubling of their serum creatinine. However, of the 2207 participants with baseline microalbuminuria, fewer receiving benazepril and amlodipine reverted to normoalbuminuria than those receiving benazepril and hydrochlorothiazide (41.7% vs 68.3%, $P = .0016$).

The Prevention of Renal and Vascular Endstage Disease Intervention Trial (PREVEND-IT) is one of the few studies specifically aimed at reducing urinary albumin excretion among otherwise healthy patients with MA.[43] Eight hundred sixty-four participants were randomized in a 2 × 2 factorial design to fosinopril 20 mg or placebo and to pravastatin 40 mg or placebo. Over 4 years of treatment, fosinopril led to a 21% reduction in urinary albumin excretion; mean systolic blood pressure initially decreased from 129 mm Hg to 124 mm Hg. By study end, however, systolic blood pressure increased to 129 mm Hg. Treatment with pravachol was not associated with a decrease in albumin excretion, despite a 24% reduction in low-density cholesterol. There was a trend toward a reduction in events with fosinopril, but no significant effect on events with pravachol. PREVEND-IT was limited by a small sample size and a lower-than-expected event rate, and therefore the question remains whether targeting MA directly leads to improved outcomes.

RELATIONSHIP BETWEEN EGFR AND MA

The few studies that have evaluated the presence of both a mildly reduced eGFR and MA suggest that they result from two distinct processes and that their relative contributions to overall risk are not the same. In the NHANES data from 1988 to 2000, only 8.3% of the participants with an eGFR 60–89 mL/min/1.73 m^2 also had MA.[2] Among participants with eGFR 60 to 89 mL/min/1.73 m^2, the RR for a CV event increased from 1.48 (95% CI 1.13 to 1.93) to 2.19 (95% CI 1.55 to 3.10) with the addition of MA; among those with MA and a normal eGFR, the RR was 2.18 (95% CI, 1.45 to 3.29), suggesting that a mildly reduced eGFR does not add significantly to overall risk in the presence of MA. Similar results were seen in observational analyses from the Action in Diabetes and Vascular disease: preterAx and diamicroN-MR Controlled Evaluation (ADVANCE) trial, which randomized participants with diabetes to a fixed combination of an ACEI and diuretic or placebo.[44] Interestingly, patients with an eGFR 30 to 59 mL/min/1.73 m^2 but without MA actually had a lower adjusted HR for a CV event (1.37, 95% CI 1.11 to 1.69) than patients with an eGFR 60 to 89 mL/min/1.73 m^2 but who also had MA (1.57, 95% CI 1.32 to 1.88).

SUMMARY

The available data about cardiovascular risk among patients with mild renal dysfunction— either by a reduction in eGFR or with the presence of MA—suggest that patients with MA are more consistently at elevated CV risk, while the significance of a reduced eGFR is more dependent on each patient's additional risk factors. The exact mechanism by which patients with mild renal dysfunction are at increased CV risk is still being explored. Patients appear to achieve significant benefit from risk factor reduction, both by medical therapy for control of chronic risk factors, and by more invasive measures, such as PCI. However, an important area of further study is whether tailoring therapy to normalize renal function reduces the risk of CV events.

REFERENCES

1. Sarnak MJ, Levey AS, Schoolwerth AC, et al. Kidney disease as a risk factor for development of cardiovascular disease: a statement from the American Heart Association Councils on Kidney in Cardiovascular Disease, High Blood Pressure Research, Clinical Cardiology, and Epidemiology and Prevention. Circulation 2003;108(17):2154–69.
2. Astor BC, Hallan SI, Miller ER 3rd, et al. Glomerular filtration rate, albuminuria, and risk of cardiovascular and all-cause mortality in the US population. Am J Epidemiol 2008;167(10):1226–34.
3. Levey AS, Coresh J, Balk E, et al. National Kidney Foundation practice guidelines for chronic kidney disease: evaluation, classification, and stratification. Ann Intern Med 2003;139(2):137–47.
4. Manjunath G, Tighiouart H, Ibrahim H, et al. Level of kidney function as a risk factor for atherosclerotic cardiovascular outcomes in the community. J Am Coll Cardiol 2003;41(1):47–55.
5. Brugts JJ, Knetsch AM, Mattace-Raso FU, et al. Renal function and risk of myocardial infarction in an elderly population: the Rotterdam Study. Arch Intern Med 2005;165(22):2659–65.
6. Kurth T, de Jong PE, Cook NR, et al. Kidney function and risk of cardiovascular disease and mortality in women: a prospective cohort study. BMJ 2009; 338:b2392.
7. Schillaci G, Pirro M, Mannarino MR, et al. Relation between renal function within the normal range and central and peripheral arterial stiffness in hypertension. Hypertension 2006;48(4):616–21.
8. Smith GL, Masoudi FA, Shlipak MG, et al. Renal impairment predicts long-term mortality risk after acute myocardial infarction. J Am Soc Nephrol 2008;19(1):141–50.
9. Anavekar NS, McMurray JJ, Velazquez EJ, et al. Relation between renal dysfunction and cardiovascular outcomes after myocardial infarction. N Engl J Med 2004;351(13):1285–95.
10. Sarafidis PA, Li S, Chen SC, et al. Hypertension awareness, treatment, and control in chronic kidney disease. Am J Med 2008;121(4):332–40.
11. Rahman M, Pressel S, Davis BR, et al. Cardiovascular outcomes in high-risk hypertensive patients stratified by baseline glomerular filtration rate. Ann Intern Med 2006;144(3):172–80.
12. Brugts JJ, Boersma E, Chonchol M, et al. The cardioprotective effects of the angiotensin-converting enzyme inhibitor perindopril in patients with stable coronary artery disease are not modified by mild-to-moderate renal insufficiency: insights from the EUROPA trial. J Am Coll Cardiol 2007;50(22):2148–55.
13. Solomon SD, Rice MM, Jablonski KA, et al. Renal function and effectiveness of angiotensin-converting enzyme inhibitor therapy in patients with chronic stable coronary disease in the Prevention of Events with ACE inhibition (PEACE) trial. Circulation 2006; 114(1):26–31.
14. Huskey J, Lindenfeld J, Cook T, et al. Effect of simvastatin on kidney function loss in patients with coronary heart disease: findings from the Scandinavian Simvastatin Survival Study (4S). Atherosclerosis 2009;205(1):202–6.
15. Shepherd J, Kastelein JJ, Bittner V, et al. Effect of intensive lipid lowering with atorvastatin on renal function in patients with coronary heart disease: the Treating to New Targets (TNT) study. Clin J Am Soc Nephrol 2007;2(6):1131–9.
16. Szummer K, Lundman P, Jacobson SH, et al. Influence of renal function on the effects of early revascularization in non-ST-elevation myocardial infarction: data from the Swedish Web System for

Enhancement and Development of Evidence-Based Care in Heart Disease Evaluated According to Recommended Therapies (SWEDEHEART). Circulation 2009;120(10):851–8.

17. Blackman DJ, Pinto R, Ross JR, et al. Impact of renal insufficiency on outcome after contemporary percutaneous coronary intervention. Am Heart J 2006; 151(1):146–52.

18. Stehouwer CD, Smulders YM. Microalbuminuria and risk for cardiovascular disease: analysis of potential mechanisms. J Am Soc Nephrol 2006;17(8):2106–11.

19. Foster MC, Hwang SJ, Larson MG, et al. Cross-classification of microalbuminuria and reduced glomerular filtration rate: associations between cardiovascular disease risk factors and clinical outcomes. Arch Intern Med 2007;167(13):1386–92.

20. Duka I, Bakris G. Influence of microalbuminuria in achieving blood pressure goals. Curr Opin Nephrol Hypertens 2008;17(5):457–63.

21. Rossi MC, Nicolucci A, Pellegrini F, et al. Identifying patients with type 2 diabetes at high risk of microalbuminuria: results of the DEMAND (Developing Education on Microalbuminuria for Awareness of reNal and cardiovascular risk in Diabetes) Study. Nephrol Dial Transplant 2008;23(4):1278–84.

22. Wachtell K, Palmieri V, Olsen MH, et al. Urine albumin/creatinine ratio and echocardiographic left ventricular structure and function in hypertensive patients with electrocardiographic left ventricular hypertrophy: the LIFE study. Losartan Intervention for Endpoint Reduction. Am Heart J 2002;143(2):319–26.

23. Palmieri V, Tracy RP, Roman MJ, et al. Relation of left ventricular hypertrophy to inflammation and albuminuria in adults with type 2 diabetes: the strong heart study. Diabetes Care 2003;26(10): 2764–9.

24. Tuttle KR, Puhlman ME, Cooney SK, et al. Urinary albumin and insulin as predictors of coronary artery disease: an angiographic study. Am J Kidney Dis 1999;34(5):918–25.

25. Solomon SD, Lin J, Solomon CG, et al. Influence of albuminuria on cardiovascular risk in patients with stable coronary artery disease. Circulation 2007; 116(23):2687–93.

26. Effects of ramipril on cardiovascular and microvascular outcomes in people with diabetes mellitus: results of the HOPE study and MICRO-HOPE substudy. Heart Outcomes Prevention Evaluation Study Investigators. Lancet 2000; 355(9200):253–9.

27. Jensen JS, Feldt-Rasmussen B, Strandgaard S, et al. Arterial hypertension, microalbuminuria, and risk of ischemic heart disease. Hypertension 2000; 35(4):898–903.

28. Gerstein HC, Mann JF, Yi Q, et al. Albuminuria and risk of cardiovascular events, death, and heart failure in diabetic and nondiabetic individuals. JAMA 2001;286(4):421–6.

29. Klausen K, Borch-Johnsen K, Feldt-Rasmussen B, et al. Very low levels of microalbuminuria are associated with increased risk of coronary heart disease and death independently of renal function, hypertension, and diabetes. Circulation 2004; 110(1):32–5.

30. Arnlov J, Evans JC, Meigs JB, et al. Low-grade albuminuria and incidence of cardiovascular disease events in nonhypertensive and nondiabetic individuals: the Framingham Heart Study. Circulation 2005;112(7):969–75.

31. Stehouwer CD, Henry RM, Dekker JM, et al. Microalbuminuria is associated with impaired brachial artery, flow-mediated vasodilation in elderly individuals without and with diabetes: further evidence for a link between microalbuminuria and endothelial dysfunction—the Hoorn Study. Kidney Int Suppl 2004;92:S42–4.

32. Cottone S, Mule G, Nardi E, et al. Microalbuminuria and early endothelial activation in essential hypertension. J Hum Hypertens 2007;21(2):167–72.

33. Stehouwer CD, Gall MA, Twisk JW, et al. Increased urinary albumin excretion, endothelial dysfunction, and chronic low-grade inflammation in type 2 diabetes: progressive, interrelated, and independently associated with risk of death. Diabetes 2002;51(4):1157–65.

34. Jager A, van Hinsbergh VW, Kostense PJ, et al. C-reactive protein and soluble vascular cell adhesion molecule-1 are associated with elevated urinary albumin excretion but do not explain its link with cardiovascular risk. Arterioscler Thromb Vasc Biol 2002;22(4):593–8.

35. Weir MR. Microalbuminuria and cardiovascular disease. Clin J Am Soc Nephrol 2007;2(3):581–90.

36. Locatelli F, Del Vecchio L, Cavalli A. Inhibition of the renin–angiotensin system in chronic kidney disease: a critical look to single and dual blockade. Nephron Clin Pract 2009;113(4):c286–93.

37. Ravid M, Lang R, Rachmani R, et al. Long-term renoprotective effect of angiotensin-converting enzyme inhibition in noninsulin-dependent diabetes mellitus. A 7-year follow-up study. Arch Intern Med 1996;156(3):286–9.

38. Ibsen H, Olsen MH, Wachtell K, et al. Does albuminuria predict cardiovascular outcomes on treatment with losartan versus atenolol in patients with diabetes, hypertension, and left ventricular hypertrophy? The LIFE study. Diabetes Care 2006; 29(3):595–600.

39. Mann JF, Schmieder RE, McQueen M, et al. Renal outcomes with telmisartan, ramipril, or both, in people at high vascular risk (the ONTARGET study): a multicentre, randomised, double-blind, controlled trial. Lancet 2008;372(9638):547–53.

40. Bakris GL, Fonseca V, Katholi RE, et al. Differential effects of beta-blockers on albuminuria in patients with type 2 diabetes. Hypertension 2005;46(6): 1309–15.

41. Jamerson K, Weber MA, Bakris GL, et al. Benazepril plus amlodipine or hydrochlorothiazide for hypertension in high-risk patients. N Engl J Med 2008; 359(23):2417–28.

42. Bakris GL, Sarafidis PA, Weir MR, et al. Renal outcomes with different fixed-dose combination therapies in patients with hypertension at high risk for cardiovascular events (ACCOMPLISH): a prespecified secondary analysis of a randomised controlled trial. The Lancet 2010;375(9721):1173–81.

43. Asselbergs FW, Diercks GF, Hillege HL, et al. Effects of fosinopril and pravastatin on cardiovascular events in subjects with microalbuminuria. Circulation 2004;110(18):2809–16.

44. Ninomiya T, Perkovic V, de Galan BE, et al. Albuminuria and kidney function independently predict cardiovascular and renal outcomes in diabetes. J Am Soc Nephrol 2009;20(8):1813–21.

Should Targeting Albuminuria Be Part of a Cardiovascular Risk Reduction Paradigm?

Adam T. Whaley-Connell, DO, MSPH[a],
Rigas G. Kalaitzidis, MD, PhD[b],*

KEYWORDS
- Albuminuria • Cardiovascular • Hypertension
- Chronic kidney disease

The presence of albumin in the urine above normal values greater than 30 mg/d or 20 mg/L is generally defined as albuminuria. Until recently, the development of albuminuria was believed to herald progression to chronic kidney disease (CKD). However, increasing data suggest that lower levels of albuminuria, or microalbuminuria, may closely correlate with endothelial dysfunction and ultimately cardiovascular disease (CVD). According to the National Kidney Foundation-Kidney Disease Outcomes Quality Initiative (KDOQI) guidelines, the term microalbuminuria refers to urinary albumin excretion (UAE) in the range between 20 and 200 μg/min (30–299 mg/d). More than 300 mg/d is clinical albuminuria or macroalbuminuria.[1] Despite the cutoff values, albuminuria is largely a continuous variable, and higher values are related to higher CVD risk. Screening for albuminuria has been recommended for hypertensive patients,[2] with or without concomitant diabetes,[3] or early chronic CKD[1] and also for the general population.[4]

This review examines the association of albuminuria with other comorbidities associated with increased cardiovascular risk and focuses on evidence regarding the reduction of albuminuria as a concept for maximizing of cardiovascular risk reduction.

ALBUMINURIA PREVALENCE AND MEASUREMENT

The prevalence of macroalbuminuria is about 1.3% and ranges from 1% in white individuals to 2.4% in African-Americans.[5] In apparently healthy individuals the prevalence of microalbuminuria is 5% to 7%.[6,7] It increases with aging[5] and is particularly common in diabetic and hypertensive patients,[8] ranging from 10% to 40%, respectively.[6,9]

Detection and screening for proteinuria in these populations are imperative in understanding CVD risk. There are several ways to measure proteinuria, including measuring the albumin concentration or urinary albumin/creatinine ratio (UACR) in a random spot urine specimen, measuring albumin concentration and simultaneously measuring creatinine clearance in a 24-hour urinary collection, and measuring albumin levels in a timed urinary collection (eg, overnight or for 4 hours).[1,3]

MECHANISMS OF THE ASSOCIATION BETWEEN ALBUMINURIA AND CVD

The mechanisms of the association between albuminuria and its link with CVD are still largely unknown and have not been completely

[a] Division of Nephrology and Hypertension, Department of Internal Medicine, Harry S Truman Veterans Affairs Medical Center, University of Missouri-Columbia School of Medicine, CE417, DC043.0, Five Hospital Drive, Columbia, MO 65212, USA
[b] Department of Nephrology, University Hospital of Ioannina, Leophoros Street, Ioannina 45500, Greece
* Corresponding author.
E-mail address: rigaska@gmail.com

Cardiol Clin 28 (2010) 437–445
doi:10.1016/j.ccl.2010.04.002

elucidated. There have been many attempts to elucidate a common mechanism that underlies the association between albuminuria/microalbuminuria and CVD.

Several putative mechanisms have been proposed (**Fig. 1**) in the development of microalbuminuria and progression of overt albuminuria. The notion that microalbuminuria is a consequence of endothelial dysfunction needs to be expanded. In recent years there has been interest in understanding the microalbuminuria consequence of damage at the level of the glomerular filtration barrier and the proximal tubule. Increased albumin filtration through increased mesangial protein trafficking damages the filtration barrier at the level of the podocyte through damage to the slit-pore diaphragm. The ultrafiltered proteins in excess are then toxic to the tubular cells, resulting in tubular damage, interstitial inflammation, and scarring.[10] Although this mechanism seems plausible, most data suggest that a constellation of pathophysiologic processes, which reflects vascular injury that results in endothelial dysfunction, chronic low-grade inflammation, or increased transvascular leakage of macromolecules, underlies the association between microalbuminuria and CVD (**Fig. 2**).[11]

Theoretically, endothelial dysfunction could contribute to albuminuria by increasing glomerular pressure and ultimately permeability.[12] The proposed mechanisms primarily involve local injury to the vascular smooth muscle and endothelial cells through oxidative stress and inflammation. Subsequent reductions in bioavailable nitric oxide and increases in a variety of proinflammatory cytokines culminant in cell proliferation and increased vascular permeability. The concept that microalbuminuria reflects a systemic vascular leakage of albumin, which might predispose to greater penetration of atherogenic lipoprotein particles into the arterial wall, is referred to as the Steno hypothesis.[12–14]

Albuminuria as an early sign of vascular injury imposed by strain vessels was recently proposed as a possible cerebrocardiorenal connection. Strain vessels are small and short perforating arteries that are exposed to high pressure and have to maintain strong vascular tone to provide large pressure gradients from the parent vessels to the capillaries. Analogous to the perforating arteries are the glomerular afferent arterioles of the juxtamedullary nephrons in the kidney. Perforating arteries exist in the central nervous system and in the retinal and coronary arteries. This process is referred to as the strain vessel hypothesis.[15]

Another possible explanation is that all the individuals may not have the same degree of endothelial function. The endothelial function is reflected by the glycocalix function, which varies genetically within normal individuals as well as by disease state. As an example, patients with type 1 diabetes are characterized by endothelial glycocalyx damage, the severity of which is increased in presence of microalbuminuria. Differences between individuals' level of albumin excretion are observed from an early age. The interindividual variability seems to be relatively constant in the first 5 decades of life, indicating that microalbuminuria is not necessarily a consequence of vascular damage at later age. Higher levels of urinary

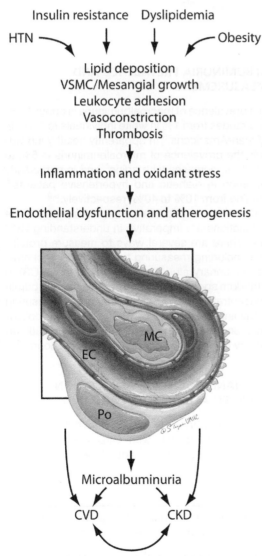

Fig. 1. Proposed mechanisms of the association between albuminuria and CVD. HTN, hypertension; MC, mesangial cell; PO, podocyte; VSMC, vascular smooth muscle cell.

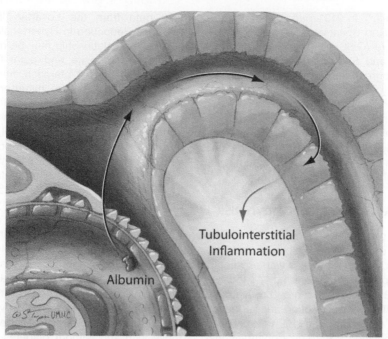

Fig. 2. Ultrafiltered proteins in excess are toxic to the tubular cells, resulting in tubular damage and interstitial inflammation in the kidney.

albumin seem to reflect the ordinary interindividual variability in endothelial function.[16]

COMORBIDITIES WITH INCREASED CARDIOVASCULAR RISK ASSOCIATED WITH ALBUMINURIA

Increases in albumin excretion are predicted by several cardiovascular risk factors, including age, glycosylated hemoglobin level, waist circumference, smoking, systolic blood pressure, and estimated glomerular filtration rate (eGFR) at baseline.[17] Several comorbidities are associated with albuminuria, such as hypertension, salt sensitivity, dyslipidemia, diabetes,[18] and heart failure,[19] all CVD risk factors that have been shown to mitigate endothelial function, oxidative stress, and inflammatory pathway, which contribute to albuminuria (see **Fig. 1**).

Hypertension is a leading cause and an important modifiable risk factor of CVD. It has been shown that higher levels of albuminuria within the normal range predict incident hypertension[20] and patients with albuminuria were less likely than patients without albuminuria to attain their systolic blood pressure goal.[21,22] The number of blood pressure medications needed to achieve the blood pressure goal has a direct correlation with the levels of proteinuria.[22]

Hypertensive patients with diabetic kidney disease who had microalbuminuria needed

a second drug to lower systolic blood pressure to less than 140 mm Hg, an observation that did not hold with those who did not have microalbuminuria.[23] Many investigators have assumed that blood pressure reduction is concordant with changes in proteinuria. There is now increasing evidence that the level of proteinuria and not GFR is most relevant for determining the future course of CKD.[24] In patients who reached the current blood pressure target, the magnitude and probability of nephropathy progression are clearly linked with the degree of proteinuria reduction.[25,26]

Increased albuminuria has also been associated with heart failure onset in various populations[19,27–29] and is considered a risk predictor of heart failure.[28,29] Almost one-third of patients with chronic systolic heart failure have albuminuria at some level. In the recent Candesartan in Heart Failure-Assessment of Mortality and Morbidity (CHARM) trial, 30% of the cohort had microalbuminuria and 11% had macroalbuminuria.[19] In this population one-third of patients without diabetes had microalbuminuria or macroalbuminuria and more than one-third of those without hypertension or renal impairment also had increased UACR, findings that cannot be explained by concomitant diabetes, hypertension, or renal dysfunction. On the other hand it was also suggested that albuminuria may be more dependent on the comorbid disease instead of heart failure itself.[30] In 2131 patients enrolled in the Gruppo Italiano Sperimentazione Streptochinasi-Heart Failure (GISSI-HF) trial 9.9% had microalbuminuria and 5.4% had overt proteinuria. There was a progressive increase in the adjusted rate of mortality in the study population in the subgroup of patients without diabetes or hypertension with increasing albuminuria.[31] The association of albuminuria with heart failure is also evident in midage nondiabetic and nonhypertensive individuals with low levels of albuminuria below the threshold for microalbuminuria.[27]

ALBUMINURIA AS A MARKER OF CVD RISK

Clinical trials provide a spectrum of results regarding the association of albuminuria, with CVD risk a clear finding in patients with or without diabetes or hypertension (**Table 1**).[32–40] Individuals with type 2 diabetes are a group at high risk for adverse CVD events, a notion supported by the association with increasing UAE that predicts CVD in this population.[41] A 10-year observational follow-up study of 939 adults with insulin-dependent diabetes mellitus suggested that increased UAE was an independent risk marker for all-cause mortality after adjustment for well-known CVD risk factors such as age, sex, socioeconomic status, hypertension, and tobacco use. The mortality in those individuals with microalbuminuria was higher than in those without but substantially lower than in patients with overt macroalbuminuria.[37] In another 5-year cohort study of 427 patients with diabetic kidney disease, all-cause mortality and CVD increased significantly and continuously across quintiles of baseline UAE. The rate of change of albuminuria in 1 year independently predicted all-cause mortality and cardiovascular mortality. A rate of change of albuminuria 30% or greater independently predicted mortality and cardiovascular events.[40]

The observation that increasing UAE predicted CVD event rate was confirmed with data from the Reduction in Endpoints in Non-Insulin Dependent Diabetes Mellitus with the Angiotensin II Antagonist Losartan (RENAAL) trial, a double-blind, randomized trial in 1513 patients with type 2 diabetes with nephropathy, focusing on the relationship between the prespecified CVD end point (composite) or hospitalization for heart failure and baseline or reduction in albuminuria. Patients with high baseline albuminuria (≥ 3 g/g creatinine) had a higher risk for the CVD end point and heart failure compared with patients with low albuminuria (<1.5 g/g).[42]

Whereas the RENAAL trial suggests a clear demarcation in the level of albuminuria and CVD risk, data from the Losartan Intervention for Endpoint Reduction in Hypertension (LIFE) study suggest the relationship may be more linear. The risk of a composite end point (CVD mortality, nonfatal myocardial infarction, nonfatal stroke) in patients with diabetes, hypertension, and left ventricular hypertrophy increased with increasing UACR. For the comparison between the lowest and highest quartiles of UACR, the adjusted hazard ratio (HR) for the composite end point increased by 2.1-fold.[34] In patients enrolled, the risk of CVD morbidity and mortality increased in a continuous fashion with no apparent thresholds or plateaux.[39]

The strongest evidence for albuminuria as a prognosticator in diabetic and nondiabetic patients may come from the Heart Outcomes Prevention Evaluation (HOPE) trial. Among more than 9000 participants in this trial, the presence of microalbuminuria increased the risk of the primary aggregate end point (myocardial infarction, stroke, or cardiovascular death) similarly in those with and without diabetes, respectively.[33] Similarly, in patients with stable CVD enrolled in the Prevention of Events with Angiotensin-Converting Enzyme Inhibition (PEACE) study,[38] an albumin/creatinine ratio (ACR) even within the normal range was associated with increased risk for all-cause and CVD mortality. Individuals with increasing microalbuminuria to macroalbuminuria compared with normal ACR increased risk for all-cause and CVD mortality, respectively. Patients with the greatest increase in ACR at the average follow-up of 34 months were at greatest risk for CVD mortality. This relationship with microalbuminuria levels and CVD risk was also true in an analysis of the Nordic Diltiazem (NORDIC) study in hypertensive patients followed for 4.5 years.[32]

In the Action in Diabetes and Vascular Disease: Preterax and Diamicron-MR Controlled Evaluation (ADVANCE) trial, treatment with a low-dose fixed combination of perindopril plus indapamide versus placebo produced a significant reduction in the incidence of a composite end point of macrovascular and microvascular events in patients 55 years and older with type 2 diabetes and at least 1 CVD risk factor. Compared with patients with normoalbuminuria, the presence of either microalbuminuria or macroalbuminuria was independently associated with higher risks for CVD mortality.[36] A change from one clinical stage of albuminuria to the next was associated with a 1.6-fold or 2-fold increase in the multivariate adjusted risk of CVD events and mortality, respectively.[35]

The association seems to be consistent in the general population as well.[6,27,43–48] In 2 population

Table 1
Association of albuminuria with cardiovascular risk

Studies	Follow-up	Patients and Ages	PEs	Albuminuria	
Rossing et al[37]	Observation follow-up study 10 y	939 patients with IDDN	All-cause and CV mortality	MA Overt nephropathy	RR 1.87 (1.03, 3.40) *P*<.05 RR 2.97 (1.68, 5.24) *P*<.01
PEACE study[38]	Follow-up study 4.8 y	2977 patients with CHD	Effect of Trandolapril therapy CVD death All-cause mortality	ACR >17µg/mg M, ACR >25µg/mg W High MA to macroalbuminuria vs lowest normal HR 1.68 (0.72, 3.93) HR 1.99 (1.08, 3.70)	*P* =.01 *P*<.001
NORDIC study[32]	Follow-up study 4.5 y	10881 patients with HPTN and 4949 with MA urine samples aged 61.2 ± 7.1 y	Diltiazem-based or diuretic-and/or β-blocker-based treatment Fatal/nonfatal MI, stroke and other CV events in patients with HPTN	MA and PEs MA HR 1.35 (1.06, 1.71)	*P*<.014
NHANES Study[43]	Prospective follow-up study 13 y	14586 participants 20 y and older	Risk of CV mortality	ACR >300 mg RR 2.42 (0.99, 5.93)	*P*<.001
Gubbio Study[44]	Follow-up study 13 y	1665 participants aged 45–64 y	Incidence of CV event	UAE ≥ 18.6 µg/min M UAE ≥ 15.7 µg/min W HR 2.15(1.33, 3.49)	
Irie et al[46]	Prospective cohort study 10 y	96,000 participants aged 40–79 y	Mortality from all CV disease	Urinary dipstick: + or more RR 1.39(1,03, 1.88) M RR 2.02(1.44, 2.83) W	
HUNT II study[45]	Follow-up study 8.3 y	9709 participants 70 y and older	Risk of CV mortality	GFR >75 mL/min/1.73 m² and MA IRR 1.98(0.67, 5.86)	

Abbreviations: CV, cardiovascular; HPTN, hypertension; IDDN, insulin-dependent diabetes mellitus; IRR, incidence rate ratio; M, men; MA, microalbuminuria; MI, myocardial infarction; PEs, primary end points; RR, risk ratio; W, women.

studies, the Gubbio study[44] and the Copenhagen County study,[47] microalbuminuria was confirmed as an important predictor of CVD outcomes. The adjusted HR was 2.15-fold and 3.10-fold greater, respectively, in patients with microalbuminuria compared with those without. In the Prevention of Renal and Vascular End Stage Disease Intervention (PREVEND) study[6] microalbuminuria was associated with a 4.7% CVD mortality in 10 years. Likewise in the nonhypertensive, nondiabetic individuals of the Framingham study, the presence of microalbuminuria above the median value was associated with a rate of incident CVD events of 8.8% in 10 years compared with a 2.9% rate in individuals with microalbuminuria below the median value.[27] In a study of a representative sample of 14,586 US adults from the general population, a doubling of albuminuria was associated with an increased incidence for CVD mortality.[43] Likewise in a prospective, population-based study of 5215 nondiabetic nonproteinuric individuals participating in the Tromso study, the association between low-grade albumin excretion, metabolic syndrome, cardiovascular morbidity, and all-cause mortality was examined. UAR was associated with CVD morbidity and all-cause mortality independent of the presence of the metabolic syndrome.[48]

ALBUMINURIA REDUCTION AND CV RISK REDUCTION

The current state of debate is whether albuminuria independent of blood pressure control or presence of prevalent CKD is truly a therapeutic target, or marker, to optimally reduce CVD risk. Assessing to what extent the effect of a therapeutic intervention aimed at preventing CVD morbidity and mortality could be explained through its incidence on the rate of UAE may prove difficult. Nonpharmacologic measures such as diet, exercise, alcohol moderation, and smoking cessation must be emphasized but are inadequate alone for management. Several interventions such as blood pressure reduction, lipid lowering, and glycemic control contribute to reductions in albuminuria and improvements in CVD prognosis. However, to our knowledge, there are no large-scale, prospective data to show that, independent of blood pressure control, a reduction in microalbuminuria results in a lower incidence of CVD events. There are retrospective data to support the hypothesis that targeting albuminuria reduction reduces the risk of subsequent CVD events.

Clinical trials provide a spectrum of results regarding the protective effects of renin angiotensin aldosteron system (RAAS) blocking agents.

Inhibition of the RAAS incorporating angiotensin-converting enzyme (ACE) inhibitors and angiotensin II receptor blockers (ARBs) not only reduces blood pressure but has significant cardio- and renoprotective effects. Treatment with agents that block the RAAS lower the risk of a composite CVD event, improve the UACR, and retard the progression from microalbuminuria to macroalbuminuria.[49,50] A diet high in sodium chloride seems to mitigate against the antiproteinuric benefit of RAAS blockade.[51]

The LIFE study[52] showed that a reduction in albuminuria during treatment was temporally associated with reductions in CVD events.[52] When UACR was reduced by 1 stratum or more, the CVD event rate reduced accordingly.[34] In the RENAAL study reducing albuminuria in the first 6 months seemed to afford cardiovascular protection. An almost linear positive relationship was found between the degree of albuminuria reduction and risk for CVD end point. Every 50% reduction in albuminuria reduces the risk for a CVD end point by 18% (95% confidence interval 9%–25%).[42] In the HOPE study treatment with an ACE inhibitor, ramipril significantly lowered the risk of the composite CVD event end point in patients 55 years and older with CVD and diabetes and at least 1 other cardiovascular risk factor (14% vs 17.8%, P<.001 vs placebo).[53] In the subgroup of diabetes population the risk of progression to overt nephropathy was reduced by 24% in ramipril recipients.[54]

The PREVEND study had a substudy that randomized 846 normotensive, nondiabetic patients without cardiovascular risk factors but with microalbuminuria to fosinopril or placebo and to pravastatin or placebo. At the end of a 4-year follow-up, fosinopril was associated with 26% reduction in UAE excretion and showed a trend towards lower CVD mortality and morbidity.[55]

The Ongoing Telmisartan Alone and in Combination with Ramipril Global Endpoint (ONTARGET) Trial was a CVD outcome study that compared ramipril with telmisartan with the combination telmisartan plus ramipril in more than 25,000 people.[56] The primary composite CVD outcome was documented in 16.5%, 16.7%, and 16.3% of ramipril, telmisartan, and a combination of the two, respectively. The incidence of the combined renal outcome (dialysis, doubling of serum creatinine, and death) was similar in recipients of either monotherapy and lower than in recipients of the combination. The combination resulted in greater blood pressure and proteinuria reduction but not lower CVD event rates.[57] Only 1000 participants of the overall trial had macroalbuminuria (<4% of the total cohort) and 300 had proteinuria greater than 1 g/g creatinine (~1.2% of the total cohort).

The question remains whether this risk reduction is explained not only by albuminuria reduction but by the concomitant reduction of high blood pressure. This situation is illustrated by data from a prospective follow-up study of 67 normotensive patients without antihypertensive treatment, with type 2 diabetes and microalbuminuria, followed for about 4.7 years and with CVD end points (eg, composite of death, CVD, cerebrovascular events, and peripheral artery disease). Patients with the reduction of albuminuria of 30% or greater were at lower risk for reaching the end point and after adjustment for sex, age, systolic blood pressure, total/high-density lipoprotein (HDL) cholesterol ratio, and current smoking in a multivariate regression model, change of albuminuria remained an independent, significant predictor.[58]

There is no consensus that proteinuria reduction independent of targeting blood pressure reduction is the primary cardiovascular risk reduction strategy, although it seems reasonable to suggest that the effect of the therapeutic intervention is difficult to assess independent of other risk factors. The implication of albuminuria in this multifactorial situation is variable and has not been completely elucidated. However, albuminuria reduction should be a CVD risk reduction paradigm even although it has still to be proved in large prospective studies.

SUMMARY

Recent advances in this field have allowed us to have a greater understanding of the epidemiology, pathophysiology, and clinical significance of albuminuria among those with or without diabetes and/or hypertension and in the general population. Routine measurement of albuminuria should be performed in high-risk patients such as those who have diabetes, hypertension, or other comorbidities or cardiovascular risk factors. Albuminuria should be considered when assessing and managing an individual's cardiovascular risk and could become a modifiable cardiovascular risk marker for cardiovascular risk reduction. Strong consideration should be given to using agents that block the RAAS as part of the regimen because they reduce albumin excretion to a greater extent than just lowering blood pressure.

REFERENCES

1. Kidney Disease Outcomes Quality Initiative (K/DOQI). K/DOQI clinical practice guidelines on hypertension and antihypertensive agents in chronic kidney disease. Am J Kidney Dis 2004;43(5 Suppl 1):S1–290.
2. Mancia G, De BG, Dominiczak A, et al. 2007 Guidelines for the Management of Arterial Hypertension: The Task Force for the Management of Arterial Hypertension of the European Society of Hypertension (ESH) and of the European Society of Cardiology (ESC). J Hypertens 2007;25(6):1105–87.
3. American Diabetes Association. Nephropathy in diabetes. 2004. Diabetes Care 2004;27:S79–84.
4. Bakris GL. Microalbuminuria. Marker of kidney and cardiovascular disease. London: Current Medicine Group; 2007.
5. Coresh J, Byrd-Holt D, Astor BC, et al. Chronic kidney disease awareness, prevalence, and trends among U.S. adults, 1999 to 2000. J Am Soc Nephrol 2005;16(1):180–8.
6. Hillege HL, Fidler V, Diercks GF, et al. Urinary albumin excretion predicts cardiovascular and non-cardiovascular mortality in general population. Circulation 2002;106(14):1777–82.
7. Romundstad S, Holmen J, Kvenild K, et al. Microalbuminuria and all-cause mortality in 2,089 apparently healthy individuals: a 4.4-year follow-up study. The Nord-Trondelag Health Study (HUNT), Norway. Am J Kidney Dis 2003;42(3):466–73.
8. Atkins RC, Polkinghorne KR, Briganti EM, et al. Prevalence of albuminuria in Australia: the AusDiab Kidney Study. Kidney Int Suppl 2004;92:S22–4.
9. Parving HH, Lewis JB, Ravid M, et al. Prevalence and risk factors for microalbuminuria in a referred cohort of type II diabetic patients: a global perspective. Kidney Int 2006;69(11):2057–63.
10. Remuzzi G, Bertani T. Pathophysiology of progressive nephropathies. N Engl J Med 1998;339(20):1448–56.
11. Deckert T, Feldt-Rasmussen B, Borch-Johnsen K, et al. Albuminuria reflects widespread vascular damage. The Steno hypothesis. Diabetologia 1989;32(4):219–26.
12. Stehouwer CD, Smulders YM. Microalbuminuria and risk for cardiovascular disease: analysis of potential mechanisms. J Am Soc Nephrol 2006;17(8):2106–11.
13. Malik AR, Sultan S, Turner ST, et al. Urinary albumin excretion is associated with impaired flow- and nitroglycerin-mediated brachial artery dilatation in hypertensive adults. J Hum Hypertens 2007;21(3):231–8.
14. Stehouwer CD, Nauta JJ, Zeldenrust GC, et al. Urinary albumin excretion, cardiovascular disease, and endothelial dysfunction in non-insulin-dependent diabetes mellitus. Lancet 1992;340(8815):319–23.
15. Ito S, Nagasawa T, Abe M, et al. Strain vessel hypothesis: a viewpoint for linkage of albuminuria and cerebro-cardiovascular risk. Hypertens Res 2009;32(2):115–21.
16. de ZD, Parving HH, Henning RH. Microalbuminuria as an early marker for cardiovascular disease. J Am Soc Nephrol 2006;17(8):2100–5.

17. Solbu MD, Kronborg J, Eriksen BO, et al. Cardiovascular risk-factors predict progression of urinary albumin-excretion in a general, non-diabetic population: a gender-specific follow-up study. Atherosclerosis 2008;201(2):398–406.

18. Danziger J. Importance of low-grade albuminuria. Mayo Clin Proc 2008;83(7):806–12.

19. Jackson CE, Solomon SD, Gerstein HC, et al. Albuminuria in chronic heart failure: prevalence and prognostic importance. Lancet 2009;374(9689):543–50.

20. Forman JP, Fisher ND, Schopick EL, et al. Higher levels of albuminuria within the normal range predict incident hypertension. J Am Soc Nephrol 2008; 19(10):1983–8.

21. Bakris GL, Fonseca V, Katholi RE, et al. Differential effects of beta-blockers on albuminuria in patients with type 2 diabetes. Hypertension 2005;46(6): 1309–15.

22. Flack JM, Duncan K, Ohmit SE, et al. Influence of albuminuria and glomerular filtration rate on blood pressure response to antihypertensive drug therapy. Vasc Health Risk Manag 2007;3(6):1029–37.

23. Duka I, Bakris G. Influence of microalbuminuria in achieving blood pressure goals. Curr Opin Nephrol Hypertens 2008;17(5):457–63.

24. So WY, Kong AP, Ma RC, et al. Glomerular filtration rate, cardiorenal end points, and all-cause mortality in type 2 diabetic patients. Diabetes Care 2006; 29(9):2046–52.

25. Eijkelkamp WB, Zhang Z, Remuzzi G, et al. Albuminuria is a target for renoprotective therapy independent from blood pressure in patients with type 2 diabetic nephropathy: post hoc analysis from the Reduction of Endpoints in NIDDM with the Angiotensin II Antagonist Losartan (RENAAL) trial. J Am Soc Nephrol 2007;18(5):1540–6.

26. Lea J, Greene T, Hebert L, et al. The relationship between magnitude of proteinuria reduction and risk of end-stage renal disease: results of the African American study of kidney disease and hypertension. Arch Intern Med 2005;165(8):947–53.

27. Arnlov J, Evans JC, Meigs JB, et al. Low-grade albuminuria and incidence of cardiovascular disease events in nonhypertensive and nondiabetic individuals: the Framingham Heart Study. Circulation 2005;112(7):969–75.

28. Arnold JM, Yusuf S, Young J, et al. Prevention of heart failure in patients in the Heart Outcomes Prevention Evaluation (HOPE) Study. Circulation 2003;107(9):1284–90.

29. Okin PM, Wachtell K, Devereux RB, et al. Combination of the electrocardiographic strain pattern and albuminuria for the prediction of new-onset heart failure in hypertensive patients: the LIFE study. Am J Hypertens 2008;21(3):273–9.

30. Smilde TD, Damman K, van der Harst P, et al. Differential associations between renal function and "modifiable" risk factors in patients with chronic heart failure. Clin Res Cardiol 2009;98(2):121–9.

31. Masson S, Latini R, Milani V, et al. Prevalence and prognostic value of elevated urinary albumin excretion in patients with chronic heart failure. Data from the GISSI-Heart Failure (GISSI-HF) Trial. Circ Heart Fail 2010;3(1):65–72.

32. Farbom P, Wahlstrand B, Almgren P, et al. Interaction between renal function and microalbuminuria for cardiovascular risk in hypertension: the nordic diltiazem study. Hypertension 2008;52(1):115–22.

33. Gerstein HC, Mann JF, Yi Q, et al. Albuminuria and risk of cardiovascular events, death, and heart failure in diabetic and nondiabetic individuals. JAMA 2001;286(4):421–6.

34. Ibsen H, Olsen MH, Wachtell K, et al. Does albuminuria predict cardiovascular outcomes on treatment with losartan versus atenolol in patients with diabetes, hypertension, and left ventricular hypertrophy? The LIFE study. Diabetes Care 2006;29(3):595–600.

35. Ninomiya T, Perkovic V, de Galan BE, et al. Albuminuria and kidney function independently predict cardiovascular and renal outcomes in diabetes. J Am Soc Nephrol 2009;20(8):1813–21.

36. Patel A, MacMahon S, Chalmers J, et al. Effects of a fixed combination of perindopril and indapamide on macrovascular and microvascular outcomes in patients with type 2 diabetes mellitus (the ADVANCE trial): a randomised controlled trial. Lancet 2007; 370(9590):829–40.

37. Rossing P, Hougaard P, Borch-Johnsen K, et al. Predictors of mortality in insulin dependent diabetes: 10 year observational follow up study. BMJ 1996;313(7060):779–84.

38. Solomon SD, Lin J, Solomon CG, et al. Influence of albuminuria on cardiovascular risk in patients with stable coronary artery disease. Circulation 2007; 116(23):2687–93.

39. Wachtell K, Ibsen H, Olsen MH, et al. Albuminuria and cardiovascular risk in hypertensive patients with left ventricular hypertrophy: the LIFE study. Ann Intern Med 2003;139(11):901–6.

40. Yuyun MF, Dinneen SF, Edwards OM, et al. Absolute level and rate of change of albuminuria over 1 year independently predict mortality and cardiovascular events in patients with diabetic nephropathy. Diabet Med 2003;20(4):277–82.

41. Dinneen SF, Gerstein HC. The association of microalbuminuria and mortality in non-insulin-dependent diabetes mellitus. A systematic overview of the literature. Arch Intern Med 1997;157(13):1413–8.

42. de ZD, Remuzzi G, Parving HH, et al. Albuminuria, a therapeutic target for cardiovascular protection in type 2 diabetic patients with nephropathy. Circulation 2004;110(8):921–7.

43. Astor BC, Hallan SI, Miller ER III, et al. Glomerular filtration rate, albuminuria, and risk of cardiovascular

and all-cause mortality in the US population. Am J Epidemiol 2008;167(10):1226–34.

44. Cirillo M, Lanti MP, Menotti A, et al. Definition of kidney dysfunction as a cardiovascular risk factor: use of urinary albumin excretion and estimated glomerular filtration rate. Arch Intern Med 2008; 168(6):617–24.

45. Hallan S, Astor B, Romundstad S, et al. Association of kidney function and albuminuria with cardiovascular mortality in older vs younger individuals: the HUNT II Study. Arch Intern Med 2007;167(22):2490–6.

46. Irie F, Iso H, Sairenchi T, et al. The relationships of proteinuria, serum creatinine, glomerular filtration rate with cardiovascular disease mortality in Japanese general population. Kidney Int 2006;69(7):1264–71.

47. Sehestedt T, Jeppesen J, Hansen TW, et al. Which markers of subclinical organ damage to measure in individuals with high normal blood pressure? J Hypertens 2009;27(6):1165–71.

48. Solbu MD, Kronborg J, Jenssen TG, et al. Albuminuria, metabolic syndrome and the risk of mortality and cardiovascular events. Atherosclerosis 2009; 204(2):503–8.

49. Parving HH, Lehnert H, Brochner-Mortensen J, et al. The effect of irbesartan on the development of diabetic nephropathy in patients with type 2 diabetes. N Engl J Med 2001;345(12):870–8.

50. Ruggenenti P, Fassi A, Ilieva AP, et al. Preventing microalbuminuria in type 2 diabetes. N Engl J Med 2004;351(19):1941–51.

51. Heeg JE, De Jong PE, van der Hem GK, et al. Efficacy and variability of the antiproteinuric effect of ACE inhibition by lisinopril. Kidney Int 1989; 36(2):272–9.

52. Ibsen H, Olsen MH, Wachtell K, et al. Reduction in albuminuria translates to reduction in cardiovascular events in hypertensive patients: losartan intervention for endpoint reduction in hypertension study. Hypertension 2005;45(2):198–202.

53. Yusuf S, Sleight P, Pogue J, et al. Effects of an angiotensin-converting-enzyme inhibitor, ramipril, on cardiovascular events in high-risk patients. The Heart Outcomes Prevention Evaluation Study Investigators. N Engl J Med 2000;342(3): 145–53.

54. Effects of ramipril on cardiovascular and microvascular outcomes in people with diabetes mellitus: results of the HOPE study and MICRO-HOPE substudy. Heart Outcomes Prevention Evaluation Study Investigators. Lancet 2000;355(9200): 253–9.

55. Asselbergs FW, Diercks GF, Hillege HL, et al. Effects of fosinopril and pravastatin on cardiovascular events in subjects with microalbuminuria. Circulation 2004;110(18):2809–16.

56. Yusuf S, Teo KK, Pogue J, et al. Telmisartan, ramipril, or both in patients at high risk for vascular events. N Engl J Med 2008;358(15):1547–59.

57. Mann JF, Schmieder RE, McQueen M, et al. Renal outcomes with telmisartan, ramipril, or both, in people at high vascular risk (the ONTARGET study): a multicentre, randomised, double-blind, controlled trial. Lancet 2008;372(9638):547–53.

58. Zandbergen AA, Vogt L, de ZD, et al. Change in albuminuria is predictive of cardiovascular outcome in normotensive patients with type 2 diabetes and microalbuminuria. Diabetes Care 2007;30(12): 3119–21.

Lower Blood Pressure Goals in High-Risk Cardiovascular Patients: Are They Defensible?

Keith A. Hopkins, MD, George L. Bakris, MD*

KEYWORDS

- Diabetes • Hypertension • Cardiovascular outcomes
- Guidelines

EPIDEMIOLOGY

Obesity and subsequent type 2 diabetes mellitus (DM) have reached epidemic proportions in economically developed countries around the world.[1] United States estimates from the *National Health and Nutrition Examination Survey* 2004–2006 population demonstrate that 23.6 million people (approximately 11%) have DM with another 57 million carrying a diagnosis of prediabetes or impaired fasting glucose.[2] In 2009, the International Diabetes Federation reported that 285 million people, 7% of the world's population over 20 years of age, have diabetes.[3]

With up to 75% of cardiovascular disease (CVD) events attributable to diabetes and hypertension, all major guidelines, including those of the National Kidney Foundation, American Heart Association, and the Seventh Report of the Joint National Committee on Prevention, Detection, Evaluation, and Treatment of High Blood Pressure, argue for more aggressive treatment goals. Specifically, in those with diabetes, coronary artery disease, or kidney disease, the recommendation is to lower blood pressure to levels below 130/80 mm Hg.[4,5] These recommendations for a lower BP goal in these specific groups were derived from retrospective data analyses that suggest a slower decline in chronic kidney disease and greater CVD risk reduction when BP is less than 130/80 mm Hg.[6] It is unclear, however, whether or not these more aggressive BP goals are defensible based on appropriately powered prospective outcome trials.

Meta-analyses of all clinical trials, to date, demonstrate that reducing BP reduces risk for stroke and coronary heart disease. None has achieved a mean BP goal of less than 130/80 mm Hg.[7] This lack of lower BP goal achievement is even true in CVD outcome trials of diabetes. In trials like the United Kingdom Prospective Diabetes Study (UKPDS)[8] and the Hypertension Optimal Treatment (HOT) trial,[9] the systolic BP (SBP) was more than 10 mm Hg higher than this lower goal. Nevertheless, a benefit occurred on CVD reduction.

One prospective study of patients with diabetes that achieved this lower BP goal in patients was the Appropriate Blood Pressure Control in Diabetes (ABCD) trial.[10] This trial demonstrated reduced CV risk but no difference between the groups with a mean SBP of 138 mm Hg versus the intensive group at 132 mm Hg. Even in this trial, the SBP was still above 130 mm Hg.

A summary of large CVD outcome trials over the past decade with the relative CVD risk reduction

The Hypertensive Diseases Unit/Section of Endocrinology, Diabetes and Metabolism, The University of Chicago Pritzker School of Medicine, 5841 South Maryland Avenue, MC 1027, Chicago, IL 60637, USA
* Corresponding author.
E-mail address: gbakris@gmail.com

Cardiol Clin 28 (2010) 447–452
doi:10.1016/j.ccl.2010.04.003
0733-8651/10/$ – see front matter © 2010 Elsevier Inc. All rights reserved.

and achieved mean SBP is presented in **Fig. 1**. It is clear that none of the trials achieved a SBP below 130 mm Hg. The definitive answer regarding whether or not lower levels of SBP further reduce CVD risk will come from the results of the Action to Control Cardiovascular Risk in Diabetes (ACCORD) trial.[11]

OUTCOME TRIALS OF RANDOMIZED BLOOD PRESSURE LEVELS
HOT

HOT was the first trial to randomize to 3 different levels of BP control and evaluate CV risk.[9] Hypertensive men and women (n = 18,790), with a mean diastolic blood pressure of 105 mm Hg and aged 50 to 80 years, were randomly assigned to lower target diastolic blood pressures less than or equal to 90 mm Hg (achieved pressure 85.2 mm Hg), less than or equal to 85 mm Hg (achieved pressure 83.2 mm Hg), and less than or equal to 80 mm Hg (achieved pressure 81.1 mm Hg). The average age (61.5 years), percentage male (53%), and percent of smokers (15.9%, 15.38%, and 15.9%) were the same across all diastolic treatment groups. Although the primary analysis failed to show a CV risk benefit of the lower BP goal, a retrospective subgroup analysis demonstrated that in the 1501 diabetic subjects, a 51% reduction in major cardiovascular (CV) morbidity (*P* = .005) occurred in the group with pressures less than or equal to 80 mm Hg compared with the group with a target pressure of less than or equal to 90 mm Hg. This risk reduction was associated with

a reduction in diastolic pressures of merely 4 mm Hg (achieved pressures of 85.2 vs 81.1). CV mortality was lower in the less than or equal to 80 mm Hg diabetic subgroup than in each of the other target groups. The lowest risk for major CV events was observed in the group with a mean achieved diastolic blood pressure of 82.6 mm Hg and at a mean SBP of 138.5 mm Hg. Therefore, although the secondary analysis was positive, it still did not prove that lower is better. Also, the study did not achieve a goal of less than 130/80 mm Hg.

UKPDS

The UKPDS prospectively examined 1148 patients with hypertension and type 2 DM for the effect of blood pressure reduction on CVD-related morbidity and mortality.[8] Patients were randomized to 2 treatment protocols: a tight group with goal pressures of less than 150/85 mm Hg and a less tight (or control/standard therapy) group with goals of less than 180/105 mm Hg with 21 predefined clinical endpoints. Mean pressure for both groups at study initiation was 160/94 mm Hg with similar percentages for smoking status (23% vs 22%), age (56.4 vs 56.5 years), presence of albuminuria (3% vs 4%), and levels of hemoglobin [Hb] A_{1C} (6.9% vs 6.8%) for the tight and less tight groups. With treatment, achieved pressures were 144/82 mm Hg and 154/87 mm Hg, respectively—values above the then recommended goals of less than 140/90 mm Hg. Hypertension-related CVD outcomes were 44% fewer

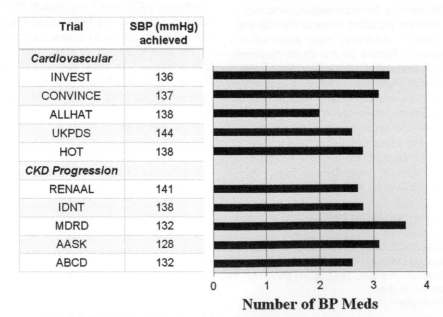

Trial	SBP (mmHg) achieved
Cardiovascular	
INVEST	136
CONVINCE	137
ALLHAT	138
UKPDS	144
HOT	138
CKD Progression	
RENAAL	141
IDNT	138
MDRD	132
AASK	128
ABCD	132

Number of BP Meds

Fig. 1. Summary of large CVD outcome trials over the past decade.

strokes (P = .013), a 21% decrease in myocardial infarction, a 56% reduction in heart failure, and a 37% decrease in the microvascular endpoints. All-cause mortality, however, was not significantly reduced. Thus, there was a clear benefit in CV outcomes even at higher pressures. A 10-year follow-up of this study, however, demonstrated no difference in outcomes between the groups as BP in the group randomized to the lower BP regressed up to the higher BP.[12] Thus, there is no BP memory with regard to CV risk reduction.

ABCD

One randomized prospective trial that closely maintained a lower BP goal in patients with diabetes was the ABCD trial.[10] Its primary hypothesis was that intensive blood pressure control would prevent or slow the progression of diabetic nephropathy, retinopathy, and CV events more than a moderate protocol. This trial of 950 patients with type 2 DM, between the ages of 40 and 74 years, had 2 treatment groups, one that had hypertension (diastolic blood pressure of 90 mm Hg) and the other normotensive (diastolic blood pressure of 80 mm Hg) at the time of randomization. SBPs were 156 mm Hg and 154 mm Hg, respectively, at baseline. Groups were randomized to receive nisoldipine or enalapril, with other medications added as needed for further blood pressure control. The trial demonstrated reduced CVD events in overall, but there was no difference in event rates between the group with a mean SBP of 138 mm Hg and the intensive group at 132 mm Hg at study's end. In the follow-up period, despite intensive treatment, both study groups demonstrated similar reduction in cardiac events as blood pressures approached but did not fall below 130/80 mm Hg. The normotensive group at baseline did maintain lower pressures, however, and although the follow-up period was not long enough, it could be argued that over a 20-year period they may do better, as the preliminary data demonstrate from this trial.[13]

Action in Diabetes and Vascular Disease: Preterax and Diamicron MR Controlled Evaluation (ADVANCE)

ADVANCE enrolled 11,140 men and women with diabetes at 215 collaborating centers worldwide.[14] The treatment groups were randomized to a combination of perindopril with indapamide or matching placebo in addition to any other current medical therapies. The average age was 66 years and average blood pressure in the whole group of 145/81 mm Hg. This is consistent with predominate systolic hypertension. Participants were required by protocol to have a history of major CVD (stroke, myocardial infarction, or hospital admission for transient ischemic attack) or at least one other risk factor for CVD. These risk factors included any level of albuminuria defined as greater than 30 mg/d or a diagnosis of type 2 DM made 10 years or more before entry. Approximately 32% of the group had a history of previous macrovascular events.

After approximately 4.3 years of follow-up, blood pressure was reduced by 5.6 mm Hg systolic and 2.2 mm Hg diastolic in the treatment group compared with those assigned to placebo. The relative risk of a major macro- or microvascular event was reduced by 9%. The relative risk of death from CVD was reduced by18%. The overall mortality risk was reduced by 14%.

In this trial, improved morbidity and mortality was shown in a cohort with lower initial blood pressures, younger age, and a wider racial demographic, but there were no data that supported the treatment goal of less than 130/80 mm Hg even though this study was appropriately powered to assess the effects of blood pressure on outcome.

Stop Atherosclerosis in Native Diabetics Study (SANDS)

SANDS enrolled 548 men and women aged 40 years or older with type 2 DM and followed them at 4 US clinical centers for CV events during aggressive treatment of blood pressure and lipid reduction in a 2-by-2 design.[15] The study evaluated CV risk markers that are associated with a higher risk of CV events in a group of hypertensive Native Americans, defined by Indian Health Service criteria with type 2 DM was studied. They specifically assessed intermediary measures of CV risk (ie, actual clinical events, common carotid artery intimal medial thickness, and carotid/cardiac ultrasonographic measures). In addition to type 2 DM, eligibility criteria also included documented low-density lipoprotein cholesterol of at least 100 mg/dL and SBPs greater than 130 mm Hg within the 12 months before randomization. The randomized BP goals were SBP of less than 115 mm Hg or less than 130 mm Hg in the aggressive and standard groups, respectively. Secondary goals were diastolic BPs of less than 75 mm Hg or less than 85 mm Hg for the 2 groups. In the aggressive therapy group, the average pressures at baseline were 128/74 mm Hg and at 36 months reduced to a mean of 117/67 mm Hg. In the standard treatment group, baseline pressures were 133/76 mm Hg and at 36 months were 129/73 mm Hg. In this high-risk, albeit younger than previous studies', cohort of patients, sustained average pressures below 130/80 mm Hg were obtained.

Primary CVD events occurred in 11 of the members of the aggressive therapy group and in 8 of the standard treatment group ($P = .51$) and the total number of CVD endpoints, primary or secondary, did not differ significantly between the 2 treatment groups. When outcomes included carotid intimal medial thickness or arterial cross-sectional area data, previously accepted markers of CVD (30), the nonsignificance of the differences did not change.

Multifactorial Intervention and Cardiovascular Disease in Patients with Type 2 DM (Steno-2)

Steno-2 looked at risk reduction in an outpatient setting of 160 patients with type 2 DM in Denmark. The endpoint of this study was death from CV causes that included strokes, myocardial infarction, and limb amputation.[16] This study was significant and different from other studies in that it evaluated the effect of multiple interventions, including exercise, dieting, and regular visits to a diabetes treatment center, along with targeted interventions on glucose, blood pressure, and cholesterol as well as the endothelial marker of inflammation, microalbuminuria in an outpatient, real world setting.

Groups were randomized to usual or intensive glucose regulation, aspirin, the use of renin-angiotensin system blockers, and lipid-lowering agents. Patients were followed for slightly more than 13 years with a mean follow-up of 7.8 years of intervention. Baseline blood pressure was 149/86 mm Hg for the conventional therapy group and 146/85 mm Hg for the intensive therapy group. The mean age at study onset was 55 years with no difference in body mass index (BMI) between the 2 groups. The initial BP goals were less than 140/85 mm Hg and less than 160/95 mm Hg for the 2 groups, respectively (1993–1999), but in 2000–2001, those goals decreased to less than 130/80 mm Hg and less than 135/85 mm Hg. At the end of the study, blood pressures were reduced by 14/12 mm Hg in the aggressive group and 3/8 in the conventional group with few serious adverse events reported in the aggressively treated group.

After 7.8 years, there was an absolute risk reduction of 20% for CVD events; the separation between the groups was noted after 4 years of therapy and was sustained over the entire course of the study. Although this study was on a homogenous cohort, the findings and process were important. It focused on multiple interventions medical and nonpharmacologic to improve outcomes.

Aggressive goals were met and markers of disease progression, such as microalbuminuria, were improved.

ACCORD

ACCORD is a large multicenter trial of 10,251 people with type 2 DM designed to test the effects of 3 different risk factor interventions on major CVD event rates.[17,18] These interventions include 2 different levels of glycemic control, lipid management to increase high-density lipoprotein cholesterol and lower triglycerides, and lastly, intensive blood pressure control randomizing to a SBP of less than 120 mm Hg or less than 140 mm Hg. Patients were randomized to receive intensive therapy (targeting HgbA$_1$C <6.0%) or standard therapy (7.0% to 7.9%). After 16 months, BP had decreased from an average of 141/76 mm Hg to 133/71 mm Hg in the standard group versus 142/76 to 120/65 mm Hg in the intensive group. At study termination, the achieved mean SBP was 112 mm Hg in the intensive group and 132 mm Hg in the conventional group.

The primary outcome is a composite of nonfatal myocardial infarction, nonfatal stroke, or death from CV causes in the vanguard population that was 52% female, 35% with a history of previous CV event, mean age 63 years, 30% African American, and 11% Latino. The mean duration of DM in these patients was 10 years. The mean HbA$_{1C}$ was 8.7%, with normal kidney function (estimated glomerular filtration rate [eGFR] 99 mL/min/1.73 m^2).

The database was locked in June 2009 but the intensive glycemic control arm was stopped in 2008, because there was a finding of higher mortality after a mean follow-up of 3.5 years.[19] Moreover, the BP arm was not stopped early for benefit or harm; thus, the results, although awaited, will probably have some caveats even if positive for the lower BP group. Thus, based on current available studies, reducing SBP to less than 130 and DBP to less than 80 cannot be safely supported.

Blood pressure is an easily obtainable biomarker for overall health.[20] Office brachial artery blood pressure may not accurately represent pressures observed by the brain, heart, and kidneys, especially in older people with predominant or isolated systolic hypertension. There is growing evidence about the importance of central artery pressures as more representative of the actual blood pressure the organs see and may be the key to lowering pressure effectively without increasing adverse events and CV risk.[21–23] A review of past outcome trials that evaluated CVD risk reduction in older high-risk people rarely achieved mean SBP below 135 mm Hg and had a difference in CV event rates. In most cases, a trend toward improved outcome is present as BP levels fall. It seems, however, that relative diastolic hypotension is the Achilles' heel of blood pressure reduction among those with predominant systolic hypertension.

Multiple post hoc analyses of outcome trials evaluating CV and renal outcomes demonstrate that lower diastolic pressures at levels below 60 mm Hg are associated with increased mortality in some cohorts,[24,25] especially those with coronary disease.[26]

In the International Verapamil-Trandolapril Study (INVEST) of 22,000 patients, all with hypertension and coronary artery disease were randomized to 2 different therapeutic regimens for hypertension and evaluated to CVD events over 3 years.[27] This cohort was had an average age of 66, 28% with diabetes and a mean BMI of 29.

The relationship between widened pulse pressures (ie, lower diastolic blood pressures) and CVD (death, myocardial infarction, or stroke) was evident in this trial. Moreover, low diastolic pressure was connected to an increased risk for myocardial infarction but not stroke.[28] INVEST participants had well-controlled SBP even in patients who had higher CVD event rates associated with low diastolic pressure. The risk for the primary outcome, all-cause death, and myocardial infarction, but not stroke, progressively increased with a diastolic pressure below 70 mm Hg (38).

A post hoc analysis of the Irbesartan Diabetic Nephropathy Trial (IDNT) also showed a J-curve relationship between CV mortality and diastolic pressure reduction in a group of patients with advanced proteinuric nephropathy with a mean eGFR of approximately 43 mL/min at baseline.[29] In this trial, risk for CV mortality started to increase at blood pressure levels less than 110/65 mm Hg.[29,30] Most events CV deaths were thought related to underlying heart failure.

SUMMARY

This review highlights the paucity of data that support actively decreasing blood pressures to a level of less than 130/80 mm Hg. Although the data support a lower CV event rate with this lower level of pressure in high-risk CV patients, early aggressive intervention to prevent levels from going above this mark would prevent development of worsening atherosclerosis. Although no trial will ever prove this concept of prevention, common sense and multiple animal experiments clear support it.

A diastolic pressure of less than 80 mm Hg is associated with a higher CV event rate in people with angina; however, the actual level in all others seems to vary between 60 and 70 mm Hg. Those at greatest risk for this diastolic J-curve are the elderly. This is where central arterial pressure is useful in helping understand how low the pressure should be. The difference between brachial and central aortic pressure is directly proportional to the magnitude of the pulse pressure; thus, the higher the pulse pressure the more likely that central aortic pressure is lower for a given brachial artery pressure.

Most patients should have their SBP reduced to levels below, not at, 140 mm Hg. For those whose physiology allows, getting the levels down to between 130 and 139 mm Hg seems supported by all the evidence. In those with isolated or predominant systolic hypertension, however, the reduction in SBP pressure should also be guided by the magnitude of diastolic pressure reduction such that levels in patients without angina do not fall below 60 mm Hg.

REFERENCES

1. Flegal KM, Carroll MD, Ogden CL, et al. Prevalence and trends in obesity among US adults, 1999–2008. JAMA 2010;303(3):235–41.
2. Danaei G, Friedman AB, Oza S, et al. Diabetes prevalence and diagnosis in US states: analysis of health surveys. Popul Health Metr 2009;7:16.
3. Shaw JE, Sicree RA, Zimmet PZ. Global estimates of the prevalence of diabetes for 2010 and 2030. Diabetes Res Clin Pract 2010;87(1):4–14.
4. Chobanian AV, Bakris GL, Black HR, et al. Seventh report of the Joint National Committee on Prevention, Detection, Evaluation, and Treatment of High Blood Pressure. Hypertension 2003;42(6):1206–52.
5. KDOQI. KDOQI clinical practice guidelines and clinical practice recommendations for diabetes and chronic kidney disease. Am J Kidney Dis 2007; 49(2 Suppl 2):S12–154.
6. Khosla N, Kalaitzidis R, Bakris GL. The kidney, hypertension, and remaining challenges. Med Clin North Am 2009;93(3):697–715.
7. Staessen JA, Li Y, Thijs L, et al. Blood pressure reduction and cardiovascular prevention: an update including the 2003–2004 secondary prevention trials. Hypertens Res 2005;28(5):385–407.
8. Tight blood pressure control and risk of macrovascular and microvascular complications in type 2 diabetes: UKPDS 38. UK Prospective Diabetes Study Group. BMJ 1998;317(7160):703–13.
9. Hansson L, Zanchetti A, Carruthers SG, et al. Effects of intensive blood-pressure lowering and low-dose aspirin in patients with hypertension: principal

results of the Hypertension Optimal Treatment (HOT) randomised trial. HOT Study Group. Lancet 1998; 351(9118):1755–62.

10. Estacio RO, Jeffers BW, Gifford N, et al. Effect of blood pressure control on diabetic microvascular complications in patients with hypertension and type 2 diabetes. Diabetes Care 2000;23(Suppl 2):B54–64.

11. Cushman WC, Evans GW, Byington RP, et al. Effects of intensive blood-pressure control in type 2 diabetes mellitus. N Engl J Med 2010;362(17):1575–85.

12. Holman RR, Paul SK, Bethel MA, et al. Long-term follow-up after tight control of blood pressure in type 2 diabetes. N Engl J Med 2008;359(15):1565–76.

13. Schrier RW, Estacio RO, Mehler PS, et al. Appropriate blood pressure control in hypertensive and normotensive type 2 diabetes mellitus: a summary of the ABCD trial. Nat Clin Pract Nephrol 2007; 3(8):428–38.

14. Patel A, MacMahon S, Chalmers J, et al. Effects of a fixed combination of perindopril and indapamide on macrovascular and microvascular outcomes in patients with type 2 diabetes mellitus (the ADVANCE trial): a randomised controlled trial. Lancet 2007; 370(9590):829–40.

15. Howard BV, Roman MJ, Devereux RB, et al. Effect of lower targets for blood pressure and LDL cholesterol on atherosclerosis in diabetes: the SANDS randomized trial. JAMA 2008;299(14):1678–89.

16. Gaede P, Vedel P, Larsen N, et al. Multifactorial intervention and cardiovascular disease in patients with type 2 diabetes. N Engl J Med 2003;348(5):383–93.

17. Buse JB, Bigger JT, Byington RP, et al. Action to Control Cardiovascular Risk in Diabetes (ACCORD) trial: design and methods. Am J Cardiol 2007; 99(12A):21i–33i.

18. Cushman WC, Grimm RH Jr, Cutler JA, et al. Rationale and design for the blood pressure intervention of the Action to Control Cardiovascular Risk in Diabetes (ACCORD) trial. Am J Cardiol 2007;99(12A):44i–55i.

19. Gerstein HC, Miller ME, Byington RP, et al. Effects of intensive glucose lowering in type 2 diabetes. N Engl J Med 2008;358(24):2545–59.

20. Giles TD. Blood pressure—the better biomarker: delay in clinical application. J Clin Hypertens (Greenwich) 2007;9(12):918–20.

21. Sharman J, Stowasser M, Fassett R, et al. Central blood pressure measurement may improve risk stratification. J Hum Hypertens 2008;22(12):838–44.

22. London GM. Brachial arterial pressure to assess cardiovascular structural damage: an overview and lessons from clinical trials. J Nephrol 2008;21(1): 23–31.

23. Westerbacka J, Leinonen E, Salonen JT, et al. Increased augmentation of central blood pressure is associated with increases in carotid intima-media thickness in type 2 diabetic patients. Diabetologia 2005;48(8):1654–62.

24. Benetos A, Safar M, Rudnichi A, et al. Pulse pressure: a predictor of long-term cardiovascular mortality in a French male population. Hypertension 1997;30(6):1410–5.

25. Messerli FH, Mancia G, Conti CR, et al. Dogma disputed: can aggressively lowering blood pressure in hypertensive patients with coronary artery disease be dangerous? Ann Intern Med 2006; 144(12):884–93.

26. Somes GW, Pahor M, Shorr RI, et al. The role of diastolic blood pressure when treating isolated systolic hypertension. Arch Intern Med 1999; 159(17):2004–9.

27. Pepine CJ, Handberg EM, Cooper-DeHoff RM, et al. A calcium antagonist vs a non-calcium antagonist hypertension treatment strategy for patients with coronary artery disease. The International Verapamil-Trandolapril Study (INVEST): a randomized controlled trial. JAMA 2003;290(21):2805–16.

28. Bangalore S, Messerli FH, Franklin SS, et al. Pulse pressure and risk of cardiovascular outcomes in patients with hypertension and coronary artery disease: an INternational VErapamil SR-trandolapril STudy (INVEST) analysis. Eur Heart J 2009;30(11): 1395–401.

29. Hunsicker LG, Atkins RC, Lewis JB, et al. Impact of irbesartan, blood pressure control, and proteinuria on renal outcomes in the Irbesartan Diabetic Nephropathy Trial. Kidney Int Suppl 2004;92:S99–101.

30. Berl T, Hunsicker LG, Lewis JB, et al. Impact of achieved blood pressure on cardiovascular outcomes in the Irbesartan Diabetic Nephropathy Trial. J Am Soc Nephrol 2005;16(7):2170–9.

The Effects of Heart Failure on Renal Function

Suneel M. Udani, MD, MPH, Jay L. Koyner, MD*

KEYWORDS

- Cardiorenal • Decompensated heart failure
- Acute kidney injury • Management • Prognosis

Increasingly, heart-kidney interactions are being recognized as fundamentally important in the prognosis of each organ individually as well as the prognosis of the overall patient. Recently, Ronco and colleagues[1] have more explicitly outlined and classified the clinical cardiorenal syndrome with 5 distinct types (**Table 1**). Although each of the subtypes has different underlying etiologies, the definition of the syndrome and the classification highlights the important interactions between the 2 organ systems and how the function of each system, itself, is dependent on the other. Further, classification highlights the importance of focusing on both organ systems when establishing a therapeutic plan, ie, one must treat both the underlying cardiac and renal dysfunction to improve the function of both organ systems.

As the cardiorenal syndrome (and its subtypes) has been defined, its incidence appears to be on the rise and the impact of organ dysfunction on long-term prognosis has been recognized.[2,3] Conventional understanding of managing patients with dual organ dysfunction has focused on treating underlying risk factors for cardiac and renal dysfunction (hypertension, diabetes, atherosclerotic disease) for prevention of chronic organ dysfunction as well as the optimization of cardiac output in acute organ dysfunction. Increasingly, the focus of optimal care has shifted toward volume management and preservation of euvolemia.[4] Accordingly, whereas treatment of chronic organ dysfunction has been well established with

existing pharmacologic therapy—with focus on blockade of the renin-angiotensin-aldosterone system (RAAS)—novel treatment strategies are being explored to identify the optimal use of vasodilators, non-RAAS neurohumoral therapy, and extracorporeal therapy.

The purpose of this article is to highlight the epidemiology of concomitant cardiac and renal dysfunction and its prognostic significance for long-term organ and patient survival. Additionally we outline evolving theories of the etiology of worsening renal function in the setting of worsening cardiac function, identify conventional and innovative therapeutic strategies to treat the syndrome, and explore novel markers of renal dysfunction in the setting of worsening cardiac function.

EPIDEMIOLOGY AND PROGNOSIS OF CHRONIC HEART FAILURE AND CHRONIC KIDNEY DISEASE

The relationship of renal function with congestive heart failure (CHF), as highlighted by type I and type II cardiorenal syndromes (CRS), is present in both chronic heart failure syndromes as well as acute decompensated heart failure (ADHF). Increasing recognition of the syndrome has revealed a growing incidence of Type I and II as well as the prognostic importance of each, ie, renal dysfunction in the setting of congestive heart failure portends an independently worse

Dr Udani was supported by 5T32DK007510-23.
Dr Koyner was supported by 5K23DK81616.
Section of Nephrology, Department of Medicine, University of Chicago, MC 5100, Room S-511, 5841 South Maryland Avenue, Chicago, IL 60637, USA
* Corresponding author.
E-mail address: jkoyner@uchicago.edu

Cardiol Clin 28 (2010) 453–465
doi:10.1016/j.ccl.2010.04.004

Table 1
Classification of the cardiorenal syndrome as defined by the acute dialysis quality initiative

Classification of Cardiorenal Syndrome	Clinical Manifestation
Type I: Acute cardiorenal syndrome	Development of acute kidney injury (AKI) in the setting of sudden worsening cardiac function
Type II: Chronic cardiorenal syndrome	Progressive renal dysfunction in the setting of chronic cardiac dysfunction
Type III: Acute renocardiac syndrome	AKI precipitating worsening cardiac function
Type IV: Chronic renocardiac syndrome	Chronic renal dysfunction leading to chronic cardiac dysfunction
Type V: Secondary cardiorenal syndrome	Worsening renal and cardiac function in the setting of underlying systemic illness

outcome compared with those with preserved renal function. Although often the more clinically apparent scenario is worsening renal function in the setting of ADHF, long-term follow-up of patients with concomitant cardiac and renal dysfunction has highlighted its significance. Ahmad and colleagues,[5] in an analysis of the SOLVD (Studies of Left Ventricular Dysfunction) study population demonstrated the impact of chronic kidney dysfunction on outcomes in heart failure. Approximately 6600 subjects were studied with an overall mortality of 23.5% over the course of the study period, 89.0% of which was determined to be related directly to cardiovascular disease. Estimated baseline glomerular filtration rate (eGFR) was a small, but statistically significant independent predictor of mortality. For each 10 mL/min lower an individual's baseline eGFR, there was a 1.064 increased risk of death (95% confidence interval [CI] 1.033–1.096). In a more recent and in-depth analysis assessing the impact of stage of kidney disease and rate of progression, Khan and colleagues[6] confirmed the prognostic importance of renal dysfunction in patients with left ventricular systolic dysfunction. Once again, using the SOLVD study population, the investigators assessed the all-cause mortality of patients stratified by eGFR. There was no difference in mortality for those with eGFR greater than 90 mL/min or between 60 and 90 mL/min; however, the risk of mortality increased significantly once baseline eGFR fell below 60 mL/min, with a hazard ratio (HR) of 1.32 for 30 to 59 mL/min and 2.54 for 15 to 29 mL/min (*P* = .004 and .0003, respectively). Rate of chronic kidney disease (CKD) progression was also an important predictor of overall mortality; in patients whose eGFR fell more than 10 mL/min/y, mortality significantly increased: for the group falling 11 to 15 mL/min/y during the study period, the HR for mortality was 2.23 and for those falling more than 15 mL/min/y,

the HR for mortality was 5.63 (*P*<.0001 for both). Not only did the finding highlight the impact of baseline CKD and progression of renal dysfunction on mortality in patients with systolic dysfunction, but it also discovered that the phenomenon is not rare, as 17% of patients had a fall in eGFR by greater than 10 mL/min/y during the study period. Further, the highest risk group for rapid progression included individuals with an eGFR of more than 90 mL/min at baseline. Thus, it appears that preserved renal function does not protect an individual with systolic dysfunction from developing worsening renal function and those who have renal dysfunction have a poorer prognosis than those with stable, preserved renal function. Similar studies with different patient cohorts have confirmed these results. Weiner and colleagues[7] evaluated the associations between baseline and change in renal function and cardiovascular events over a 3-year period in a community-based population combining the Atherosclerosis Risk in Communities (ARIC) cohort and the Cardiovascular Health Study (CHS) cohort. In total, approximately 18,000 patients were studied and were stratified into 4 groups by baseline eGFR less than or greater than 60 mL/min that remained within that range for the study period or individuals who started with an eGFR greater than 60 mL/min whose eGFR fell to less than 60 mL/min and the converse. A total of 891 subjects had a stable eGFR of less than 60 mL/min, 278 subjects had an increase in their eGFR from less than 60 mL/min to more than 60 mL/min, 972 subjects had a fall in their eGFR from more than 60 mL/min to less than 60 mL/min, and the remainder had a sustained eGFR higher than 60 mL/min throughout the study period. The authors discovered that patients with the highest cardiovascular morbidity risk were the individuals with a sustained eGFR less than 60 mL/min (HR = 3.66, 95% CI 3.12–4.30). Further, the investigators discovered that either a fall in eGFR during the study period to below 60 mL/min *or* an initial eGFR below 60 mL/min and a subsequent increase above 60 mL/min during the study period carried an added risk (HR 2.48, 95% CI 2.08–2.95 and HR 2.10, 95% CI 1.50–2.92), suggesting the presence of abnormal renal function, even with some degree of variability where there is biochemical improvement, is associated with increased cardiovascular morbidity. The findings, however, did not differentiate between cardiovascular outcomes related to heart failure versus coronary artery disease or cerebrovascular disease. Nevertheless, the findings confirm the significant association of small decrements in renal function with cardiovascular morbidity even when renal function may transiently improve, and perhaps points to a flaw in the utility of eGFR as a surrogate for renal function.

The phenomenon does not appear to be limited to Western societies. In an analysis of the Japanese Cardiac Registry of Heart Failure in Cardiology (JCARE-CARD), investigators demonstrated similar long-term outcomes in Japanese patients with CKD hospitalized with heart failure. The JCARE-CARD followed a cohort of approximately 2000 patients after their hospitalization for a mean of 2.4 years and demonstrated that CKD (defined by eGFR <60 mL/min by Modification of Diet in Renal Disease [MDRD] equation) was prevalent among the study population (70.3%), and carries increased morbidity and mortality.[8] The composite end point (all-cause mortality and rehospitalization for heart failure) increased with worsening renal function (HR 1.520 and 2.566 for eGFR 30–59 mL/min and <30 mL/min, respectively as compared with eGFR >60 mL/min; P values for both <.001). Of note, patients with renal dysfunction (eGFR <60 mL/min) were also less likely to be prescribed angiotensin-converting enzyme (ACE) inhibitors, angiotensin receptor blockers (ARB), and β-blockers upon hospital discharge than those with preserved renal function—but it deserves noting that less than 50% of patients in each group were prescribed any of the medications established to improve mortality in patients with heart failure. Recent literature has confirmed the findings of earlier studies that the presence of renal dysfunction in the setting of heart failure is associated with adverse outcomes over extended, out-of-hospital follow-up. The recent findings have highlighted that smaller decrements in renal function, even transient, are similarly associated with poorer outcomes in patients with heart failure and this association transcends European and American populations.

Acute Decompensated Heart Failure and Worsening Renal Function

Previous studies have confirmed the impact of worsening renal function (WRF) or acute kidney injury in the setting of acute decompensated heart failure on length of hospitalization. In a study of approximately 300 European patients hospitalized with ADHF, approximately one-third of the patients developed WRF (72 of 248 individuals included in analysis). The presence of WRF did not appear to have an impact on overall mortality, but did have an impact on extended hospital stay.[9] However, more recent literature has identified that the WRF has broader impact than simply extending hospitalization. Rather, WRF, even if its presence is transient, independently predicts a poorer clinical outcome.

Metra and colleagues,[10] in a study of 318 consecutive patients admitted with ADHF, demonstrated the impact of worsening renal function on mortality. There were 107 patients who developed WRF, defined by an absolute increase in serum creatinine (SCr) of 0.3 mg/dL or a ≥25% increase from the admission value. Importantly, the study's intention was to identify patients who developed WRF through the course of standard heart failure therapy. The study population, thus, included patients hospitalized with acute heart failure syndromes, however excluded patients who "developed complications or underwent procedures which may cause a rise in S-Cr." Specifically, patients with a cardiac arrest, shock, or cardiac surgery or who underwent invasive procedures requiring intravenous contrast administration were excluded. After a mean follow-up period of approximately 480 days, patients who experienced WRF in the hospital had a significantly higher rate of the primary outcome—urgent hospitalization for heart failure or cardiovascular mortality with an HR of 1.47 (95% CI 1.13–1.81; P = .024).

Logeart and colleagues[11] discovered similar findings in a study of a similar patient population of 416 individuals hospitalized with acute heart failure. As in the study performed by Metra and colleagues[10] described in the preceding paragraph, individuals with cardiogenic shock, in-hospital death, and severe low-output heart failure requiring ionotropes were excluded. Also, patients with advanced CKD with a SCr greater than 230 μmol/L (approximately 2.6 mg/dL) were excluded in an attempt to include only patients where the WRF was directly related to ADHF. Despite the strict exclusion criteria, the investigators also discovered a high incidence of WRF, 152 (36.3%) of 416 patients, with WRF defined as an increase in SCr of 25 μmol/L (approximately 0.3 mg/dL). Despite a shorter follow-up period than the previous study described, the investigators also found WRF to be an independent risk factor for their primary outcome—rehospitalization for ADHF or all-cause mortality with a hazard ratio of 1.48 (95% CI 1.20–2.82, P = .01). Importantly, the study included patients whose renal function improved during the course of their hospitalization as those with WRF. Thus, the authors concluded that despite improvement, the mere presence of WRF in the setting of ADHF portends a poor prognosis.

The recent literature highlights important updates in the association between WRF and ADHF. First, in concordance with literature in other clinical settings, small increases in SCr (50% increase or absolute increase of 0.3 mg/dL from baseline as in stage I AKI as defined by the Acute Kidney Injury Network), previously thought to be of questionable clinical importance, are independently associated with both short-term and long-term clinically important outcomes.[12–15] Further, even when the small changes in SCr are transient and renal function "improves," patients' clinical prognosis remains worse than those whose renal function remains intact throughout their hospital stay.

Etiology

The natural question resulting from this finding is what are the underlying clinical or patient characteristics that lead to WRF in the setting of ADHF? Given that even transient WRF in individuals hospitalized with ADHF have worse outcomes, this suggests that the worse outcomes cannot be related only to presence of renal dysfunction, but suggests that the presence of heart failure or other aspects of the clinical milieu of patients developing WRF is different.

The studies outlined give some insight into the differences in patient characteristics associated with WRF. Specifically, in the population studied by Metra and colleagues[10] individuals with WRF were more likely to have preexisting renal dysfunction (36% vs 19%, P = .002), rales above the lung bases on auscultation (67% vs 46%, P = .001), presence of increased jugular venous pressure (41% vs 26%, P = .009), and, on echocardiography, lower mean ejection fraction (31.4% vs. 36.0%, P = .007), greater likelihood of left ventricular dilation (79% vs. 65%, P = .001), higher mean pulmonary artery pressure (47 mm Hg vs 43 mm Hg, P = .004), and a greater likelihood of a having a restrictive pattern of filling (50% vs 35%, P = .015). In contrast, in the population studied

by Logeart and colleagues[11] left ventricular ejection fraction, the sole echocardiographic data reported, did not differ between those who did and did not develop WRF. Rather, individuals developing WRF were more likely to be older, have baseline renal dysfunction, a history diabetes mellitus, a history of hypertension, lower baseline hemoglobin (mean 12.1 g/dL vs 13.1 g/dL) and hypertensive crisis (systolic blood pressure ≥ 200 mm Hg) as a precipitating cause of heart failure decompensation.[11] Thus, while recognizing differences between the groups, the identified characteristics offer limited insight into the etiology of WRF in ADHF outside of presence of baseline renal dysfunction. Further, although the concept of arterial underfilling is often used to explain WRF in the setting of ADHF, systolic and diastolic blood pressure, the presumed manifestation of hypoperfusion and arterial underfilling, did not differ between the groups in either study.[10,11] A study by Mullens and colleagues[16] with invasive monitoring of 145 patients admitted with ADHF offered additional information about characteristics of patients developing WRF with a suggestion of a biologic explanation as well. Consecutive patients admitted with ADHF underwent invasive monitoring with a pulmonary artery catheter. Similar to the previous studies outlined, WRF was defined as an increase in SCr by 0.3 mg/dL and was common (occurring in 40% of subjects). Once again renal dysfunction on admission was the only baseline difference between the 2 groups. Investigators assessed admission systolic blood pressure, cardiac index (CI), pulmonary capillary wedge pressure (PCWP), pulmonary artery systolic pressure, and central venous pressure (CVP). Only mean central venous pressure was predictive of WRF with a mean CVP 18 ± 7 mm Hg in the group developing WRF versus 12 ± 6 mm Hg, P<.001 in the group without WRF. Further, cardiac output, which is often considered to be the focus of optimized ADHF therapy, was actually *higher* in the group developing WRF (mean CI 2.0 vs 1.8, P = .008). The study investigators concluded that, perhaps, rather than arterial underfilling as the central physiologic derangement leading to WRF in ADHF, venous congestion is the primary culprit—similar to the development of cardiac cirrhosis in patients with chronic heart failure. Other investigators, in a reanalysis of data from the ESCAPE trial[17] and an investigation by Damman and colleagues[18] have discovered similar findings.

The effect of increased renal venous pressure to reduce renal blood flow, decrease single-nephron GFR, and decrease urinary sodium excretion has been well recognized in previous animal studies.

Specifically, Wathen and Selkurt[19] outlined the relationship between increases in renal venous pressure, creatinine clearance, urine volume, and urinary sodium excretion in the setting of saline loading. Once dogs were loaded with intravenous saline, renal venous pressure was increased by partial occlusion of the renal vein. Increased renal venous pressure was associated with decreased creatinine clearance, urine volume, and urinary sodium excretion as compared with dogs where renal venous pressure was left unaffected. Importantly, this occurred only in the dogs that were salt-loaded and not those who were *truly* volume depleted via removal of access to food and water for 24 hours. Burnett and Cox[20] demonstrated similar findings in their experiments. Once again, they compared the effect of increasing renal venous pressure on urinary sodium excretion and glomerular filtration rate in dogs that were restricted from any food for 24 hours before the experiment. Urinary sodium excretion, renal blood flow, and GFR were compared between the dogs before and after administration of 5% body weight of parenteral saline solution. As discovered in the study outlined previously, the saline expanded and the "hydropenic" dogs behaved differently with increases in renal venous pressure. Increases in renal venous pressure decreased urinary sodium excretion, GFR, and renal blood flow. Importantly, this study also included measures of renal interstitial pressure. Renal interstitial pressure increased to a much greater degree in the saline-expanded state for the same degree of increase in renal venous pressure than the "hydropenic" state. Thus, it appears that the effect of increased venous pressure on single-nephron GFR, urinary sodium excretion, and renal blood flow vary depending on the organism's state of sodium balance; with interstitial pressure mediating this effect. These experiments, although performed in dogs, give a putative mechanism for the clinical manifestations seen in ADHF and identified in the trials outlined earlier in this article. Although not definitive proof, it provides direction for future investigation on the link between worsening renal function and decompensated heart failure.

A similar, yet distinct, potential mechanism for WRF in the setting of ADHF is mediated by the effect of decompensated heart failure on intra-abdominal pressure. The importance of intra-abdominal pressure on renal function in the critically ill (eg, trauma, acute pancreatitis, decompensated liver disease) has been increasingly recognized. In a recent single-center study of critically ill patients, those with acute renal failure were twice as likely to have intra-abdominal hypertension than those without.[21] Similarly,

in a separate single-center study of critically ill patients with sepsis, increasing intra-abdominal pressure correlated with higher peak SCr, abdominal perfusion pressure was inversely correlated with peak SCr, and individuals with abdominal compartment syndrome (defined by intra-abdominal pressure >20 mm Hg and organ dysfunction) had a significantly higher SCr.[22]

Congestive heart failure has also been recognized as a clinical scenario where the effect of intra-abdominal pressure may be important. In a single-center study of 40 consecutive patients admitted to a heart failure unit with intra-abdominal pressure monitoring, patients with increased intra-abdominal pressure (≥ 8 mm Hg) had a higher baseline SCr (on admission) than those with lower intra-abdominal pressures. Further, changes in intra-abdominal pressure were directly proportional to changes in renal function (as measured by creatinine clearance).[23] The data do not provide a causative relationship; nevertheless, the findings do suggest a relationship among ADHF, WRF, and increased intra-abdominal pressure. A potential causative link is suggested by a separate study conducted by the same investigators on the effect of fluid removal on increased intra-abdominal pressure and renal function in the setting of ADHF. Nine patients with elevated intracardiac filling pressures, severe systolic dysfunction (left ventricular ejection fraction [LVEF] <30%), and with failure of response to medical therapy (as determined by attending cardiologist) were treated with fluid removal via paracentesis or continuous ultrafiltration. Mean intra-abdominal pressure was elevated before fluid removal (13 mm Hg). After fluid removal, the mean intra-abdominal pressure fell to 7 mm Hg. All patients had an increase in SCr after admission to the heart failure unit before fluid removal and had a significant fall in SCr after fluid removal (mean SCr 3.4 mg/dL before fluid removal and 2.4 mg/dL after fluid removal; $P = .01$).[24] Although there is not a definitive link between the mechanical removal of fluid and the change in SCr, the findings do suggest that intra-abdominal pressure is the determinant of changes in renal function in the patients with ADHF and increased intra-abdominal pressure. The investigators theorize that the benefit observed in patients with mechanical fluid removal was mediated by amelioration of renal "tamponade" physiology. Before fluid removal, the kidney existed in a state bordering on ischemia resulting in worsening renal function. Fluid removal increased abdominal perfusion pressure, thus improving renal perfusion pressure. The clear limitations of the theory are that they are founded on experience solely published from a single center and single heart failure unit. Further, no other indices are reported as surrogates for renal blood flow or renal perfusion. Specifically, neither urinary sodium excretion nor urinary urea excretion is reported as possible confirmation of the effect of fluid removal to ameliorate a state of renal ischemia. Nevertheless, the findings offer additional insight and an alternative pathway on how decompensated heart failure leads to WRF.

Highlighting the effects of venous congestion and increased intra-abdominal pressure on renal function has offered novel perspectives on the phenomenon of WRF in ADHF. Although the theories remain to be definitely proven, they have sound foundations in observed renal physiology and offer new targets for monitoring as well as therapeutic intervention. Most importantly, the theories offer alternatives to the conventional theories of "over-diuresis" and "inadequate cardiac output" that have led to misguided interventions including deleterious use of volume expansion and vasoactive drugs when alternative strategies may have been more effective.

Importantly, the mechanisms appear to contribute to WRF in the setting of an *acute* worsening of heart failure. WRF in the setting of chronic heart failure syndromes is even less clear. WRF may be attributable to chronic hypoperfusion, venous congestion, or intra-abdominal hypertension, or, simply, a concomitant manifestation of the underlying disease processes that have led to the cardiac dysfunction are unclear.

MANIFESTATIONS OF WORSENING RENAL FUNCTION

In the previously mentioned studies, evaluating patients with concomitant cardiac and renal dysfunction, SCr, and eGFR, calculated by the modified MDRD equation, are used to monitor renal function. However, SCr has clear limitations. Given its dependence on muscle mass, SCr-based estimations of renal function can underestimate or overestimate renal function at the extremes of age and body size. Further, the kidney's ability to hyperfilter in the setting of early renal injury can hide the evidence of true renal injury when tubular or glomerular damage has already begun. The finding that patients with chronic heart failure have microalbuminuria in the setting of SCr slightly above the normal range suggests that more renal damage is present than suggested by SCr.[25]

Novel biomarkers of renal function, specifically serum cystatin C and serum and urine Neutrophil Gelatinase Associated Lipocalin (NGAL), have been studied in the evaluation of both acute and chronic changes in renal function.[26,27]

Additionally, these markers have been investigated in the setting of heart failure. Poniatowski and colleagues[28] measured serum cystatin and serum and urine NGAL in 150 patients with known coronary artery disease and variable ejection fraction and New York Heart Association (NYHA) functional class without preexisting kidney disease (denoted by elevated SCr). Both serum NGAL and cystatin C increased as NYHA functional class worsened and ejection fraction decreased, with statistically significant mean value differences for NYHA class III versus class I (no class IV individuals were studied). Urinary NGAL also increased with worsening NYHA functional status class; differences were noted between class II and class I as well as class III and class I heart failure. Urine NGAL, serum creatinine, and eGFR (MDRD) were statistically significantly higher in patients with NYHA class III versus class I heart failure. The utility of urinary NGAL has been investigated in the setting of stable heart failure. Ninety patients with known CHF were compared with 20 age- and sex-matched controls with regard to SCr, eGFR, and urinary NGAL. Urinary NGAL was significantly higher in the individuals with congestive heart failure and concentrations correlated with SCr, eGFR, and N-terminal brain natriuretic peptide (NT-BNP). These study findings confirm the ability of serum NGAL and cystatin C to correspond with renal function in patients with chronic congestive heart failure. Further, it appears the markers correspond better with functional status than creatinine alone. However, it does not appear that the serum markers are superior to MDRD-based eGFR equations. Urinary NGAL, however, does appear to have added sensitivity in detecting worsening functional class before significant changes in serum creatinine or eGFR. More importantly, the elevations in serum and urinary NGAL suggest that the changes in renal function manifested by changes in urinary sodium excretion, single-nephron GFR, and creatinine clearance are not merely manifestations of purely reversible hemodynamic derangements. Given that NGAL has been demonstrated to serve as a marker of true tubular injury, its elevation in the urine suggests that renal tissue injury occurs and is ongoing in the setting of chronic heart failure. The conclusion suggests that all changes in renal function observed in patients with chronic heart failure, even in the absence of concomitant hypertensive and/or diabetic nephrosclerosis will not ameliorate simply with improvement in heart failure. Whether NGAL (or other markers of tubular injury) have value in longitudinal studies of patients with chronic heart failure and reflect intermittent decompensations and improvements in functional status remains to be studied.

Serum NGAL appears to demonstrate a similar pattern in patients with acute heart failure as in patients with chronic heart failure. In a nested analysis of patients enrolled in the Optimal Trial In Myocardial infarction with Angiotensin II Antagonist Losartan (OPTIMAAL), patients were randomized to received either captopril or losartan following a myocardial infarction that was complicated by heart failure. In these 236 subjects, serum NGAL levels were elevated initially and fell significantly after the initial hospitalization. Similar to the studies outlined previously, serum NGAL corresponded to mean NYHA functional class over the follow-up period as well as the NYHA functional class determined at the end of the follow-up period (median 2.7 years).[29]

The limitation in measurement of serum NGAL alone is that NGAL is not kidney-specific. Therefore, although elevations in serum or urine NGAL suggest possible renal tubular injury, it may be, rather, an indicator of extra-renal tissue injury. The search for the perfect kidney injury biomarker continues both for states of congestive heart failure and noncardiac causes of kidney injury. NGAL and cystatin C have demonstrated promise, but their full clinical utility remains to be determined.

TREATMENT
Treatment of Chronic Heart Failure

Although the treatment of chronic heart failure as a whole is beyond the scope of this article, the agents that are particularly applicable to renal function (and changes in renal function) are those that effect the renin-angiotensin-aldosterone axis. The positive effect of ACE inhibitors and angiotensin II receptor blockers (ARB) on cardiac function and mortality in patients with heart failure has been well established.[30–32] Despite their known beneficial effects in patients with heart failure, ACE inhibitors and ARBs remain underprescribed.[33,34] Further, renal failure remains a commonly identified reason for not prescribing ACE inhibitors or ARBs.[33,35] Therefore, the question arises, should ACE inhibitors and ARBs be used in patients with heart failure and CKD? Further, what is the appropriate response if the SCr increases with use of an ACE inhibitor or ARB?

Both the CONSENSUS (a randomized controlled trial demonstrating the benefit of enalapril on symptoms and survival in NYHA class IV heart failure) and CHARM (a randomized controlled trial demonstrating the benefit of candesartan on survival in congestive heart failure) trials

included individuals with renal dysfunction; however, the effect of treatment on these groups was not addressed specifically. Limited data are available regarding the specific use of ARBs or ACE inhibitors in patients with chronic kidney disease and heart failure. Using the database from the Digitalis Investigation Group, a randomized trial of digoxin for individuals with systolic heart failure, individuals with CKD, defined by SCr greater than 1.3 mg/dL in women and 1.5 mg/dL in men, a propensity score based on the analysis of the effect of ACE inhibitors on outcomes in heart failure in patients with CKD was created. Approximately 1700 individuals were identified and those taking ACE inhibitors were matched by propensity score with those not taking ACE inhibitors. Ultimately, 208 individuals with CKD on ACE inhibitors were studied. After adjusting for covariates and propensity score, individuals taking ACE inhibitors had a lower risk of death at 2 years (HR 0.58, 95% CI 0.35–0.96), and were less likely to have hospitalizations for decompensated heart failure (HR 0.69, 95% CI 0.48–0.90).[36] Although the propensity score based analysis and matching attempts to control for the possible confounding, the study findings are limited by the nonexperimental nature of the study.

Similarly, although not a study directly designed to study the use of ARBs in the setting of CKD and CHF, a secondary analysis of the Valsartan in Heart Failure Trial (Val-HeFT) database offers some additional insight on potential benefits of RAAS blockade. The study enrolled approximately 5100 individuals with stable, symptomatic heart failure with an ejection fraction less than 40%. The individuals were then classified according to the presence of CKD (eGFR <60 mL/min) and/or proteinuria (1+ dipstick or more). All individuals were randomized to treatment with Valsartan or placebo. Importantly, individuals with baseline SCr greater than 2.5 mg/dL were excluded. Valsartan had no effect on mortality (vs placebo) in individuals with or without CKD; however, in individuals with CKD, valsartan extended the time to first morbid event (death, sudden death with resuscitation, hospitalization for heart failure, use of vasodilators and/or ionotropes for at least 4 hours without hospitalization).[37] The limited studies suggest that the benefits of ACE inhibitors and ARBs in heart failure carry over to patients with CKD. Nevertheless, individuals with more advanced renal dysfunction were excluded from the reanalyzed studies. Until further data are available, the use of ACE inhibitors or ARBs for the indication of chronic heart failure must be individualized.

The hemodynamic effects of ACE inhibitors and ARB on the intraglomerular circulation are well described and remain a primary reason for their use in patients with chronic kidney disease. However, a common association is seen between initiation of ACE inhibitors and rise in SCr or fall in eGFR. An increase in SCr up to 30% is often seen after initiation and is associated with long-term stability of renal function.[38] Thus, an increase in SCr of 30% or less is not associated with long-term renal damage and warrants continued use of the drug in the absence of other adverse effects. A greater than 30% increase is not as reassuring and is suggestive of a state of angiotensin-dependent glomerular perfusion such as volume depletion or severe renal atherosclerotic disease and warrants discontinuation of the drug.

Direct renin inhibitors

The well-established benefit of ACE inhibitors and ARBs have led physicians to seek additional benefit in the therapy of heart failure with other means of RAAS blockade. Direct renin inhibitors (DRIs) offer an alternative as well as a complementary therapy for complete RAAS blockade. Theoretically, the use of ACE inhibitors or ARBs up-regulate renin activity to the degree where increased renin activity can overcome the effect of ACE inhibitors or ARBs and lead to continued RAAS activity. The clinical effect of DRIs on patients with heart failure, however, is not well known. McMurray and colleagues[39] studied the effect of DRIs on clinical and biologic parameters including plasma BNP (brain natriuretic peptide) and NT-BNP (N-terminal brain natriuretic peptide) in patients with NYHA Class II–IV heart failure, history of hypertension and stable use of β-Blockers, and ACE inhibitor (or ARB). A total of 296 individuals were randomized to 150 mg of aliskiren or placebo. At baseline, patients were well matched according to demographic, clinical, and biologic parameters. After 12 weeks of follow-up, individuals receiving aliskiren had a mean fall in NT-BNP 244 ± 2025 pg/mL versus a mean increase in NT-BNP of 762 ± 6123 pg/mL in the individuals receiving placebo ($P = .0106$). BNP fell in both groups, although more in the aliskiren group (61 ± 257 pg/mL vs 12.2 ± 243 pg/mL). No statistically significant differences were seen in any clinical or echocardiographic parameters or adverse events between the groups. The results of the study suggest that the use of DRIs in addition to existing, standard of care therapy for heart failure is well tolerated. Although there appear to be neurohumoral benefits, whether this translates to short- or long-term clinical benefit requires further investigation.

Aldosterone antagonists

Despite the use of ACE inhibitors or ARBs, aldosterone levels remain elevated in patients with chronic heart failure, leading physicians to explore and discover the benefits of aldosterone antagonists. The Randomized Aldactone Evaluation Study (RALES) randomized 1663 patients with severe congestive heat failure (ejection fraction < 35% and NYHA class III or IV) to an aldosterone antagonist, aldactone, versus placebo. The patients receiving aldactone had a significantly lower risk of death than the placebo group (relative risk 0.70, 95% CI 0.60–0.82).[40] The Eplerenone Post-Acute Myocardial Infarction Heart Failure efficacy and survival Study (EPHESUS) investigated the effect of an alternate aldosterone antagonist, eplerenone, on patients with left ventricular dysfunction (ejection fraction <40%) after an acute myocardial infarction with clinical signs of heart failure. Approximately 6600 individuals were randomized to eplerenone versus placebo. Similar to the RALES study, the individuals receiving the aldosterone antagonist had a lower risk of death (relative risk 0.85, $P = .008$).[41] These 2 landmark trials expanded the use of aldosterone antagonists to patients with advanced heart failure. The question remains, is their use safe and effective in patients with renal dysfunction? Importantly, in both studies, individuals with baseline SCr greater than 2.5 mg/dL were excluded. Further, the hyperkalemic effect of aldosterone antagonists was increasingly recognized after the results of the RALES study. Both the RALES and EPHESUS study excluded patients with baseline serum potassium greater than 5.0 mmol/L and individuals were closely monitored for hyperkalemia. In the RALES study, the risk of hyperkalemia was minimal (<2%) with no difference between the treatment and placebo groups. However, the widespread use of aldosterone antagonists led to much more significant hyperkalemia. After the publication of the RALES study, the rates of hyperkalemia requiring hospitalization increased from 2.4 per 1000 to 11 per 1000 in a population-based analysis of patients with a history of heart failure treated with ACE inhibitors from the province of Ontario, Canada.[42] The effect renal dysfunction had on the increased incidence of hyperkalemia remains unclear. Nevertheless, the findings question the safety and indication for aldosterone antagonists in heart failure, especially those with CKD or borderline potassium levels.

Minimal data are available to guide clinicians on the use of aldosterone antagonists in CKD to improve cardiovascular outcomes. Although not studied in patients with overt heart failure, British investigators evaluated the effect of spironolactone on left ventricular mass and aortic stiffness in patients with stage II and stage III CKD. Importantly, the inclusion criteria were individuals already being treated with ACE inhibitors, making the population as close to a "real-world" sample as possible. Left ventricular (LV) mass was determined by magnetic resonance imaging. Aortic pulse wave velocity (APWV) was measured by sequential carotid and femoral artery waveforms. A total 112 patients were studied and followed for 40 weeks including a 4-week open-label run-in period. Compared with placebo, individuals treated with spironolactone had a significant decrease in mean LV mass as well as a decrease in prevalence of LVH (-14 ± 13 g vs 3 ± 11 g, $P<.01$ for spironolactone vs placebo). Aortic pulse wave velocity decreased and aortic distensibility increased as well in the spironolactone group. After randomization, only 2 patients in the spironolactone group had hyperkalemia (serum potassium 5.5–5.9 mmol/L) requiring modification to alternate day therapy. Serum potassium in the spironolactone group at the end of the study was slightly higher than the placebo group 4.6 ± 0.6 mmol/L vs 4.4 ± 0.4 mmol/L ($P<.05$).[43] The results of the study suggest that, in a carefully selected and monitored population, aldosterone antagonists are safe and can be effective in improving some early anatomic and physiologic parameters of cardiovascular function. Importantly, the physiology of patients with CKD without systolic dysfunction may be very different from the population studied. In individuals with symptomatic heart failure much more reliant on single-nephron GFR for renal function, the hyperkalemia resulting from administration of aldosterone antagonists may be much more marked. Further, patients with diabetes, who often have coexisting renal and cardiovascular disease, were excluded from the study population. If individuals with diabetes have coexistent hypo-renin hypo-aldosteronism and type IV renal tubular acidosis physiology, the administration of aldosterone antagonists may have much more deleterious consequences, specifically increasing the rates of hyperkalemia. Nevertheless, the study provides promise that the early anatomic and physiologic changes seen in CKD that often lead to overt heart failure may be intervened upon with the use of aldosterone antagonists.

Treatment of Acute Heart Failure

As outlined, worsening renal function in the setting of acute heart failure syndromes not only is common, but also has significant effects on short- and long-term prognosis. The optimal treatment of ADHF involves addressing 2 goals: restoration of euvolemia and preservation of end-organ (including renal) function. Although the full scope of the treatment of acute heart failure is beyond the scope of this article, 2 treatment options will be reviewed as they have specific pertinence to the prevention of WRF in the setting of ADHF: ultrafiltration and the use of novel vasodilators.

The use of ultrafiltration has become increasingly popular in the treatment of ADHF primarily because of diuretic resistance as well as the increasing recognition of venous congestion as an important determinant of WRF. Despite its increasing use, minimal data exist to determine the exact short-term and long-term effects of ultrafiltration on renal function in ADHF. The available data on ultrafiltration have demonstrated its effectiveness as a tool for volume removal; however, the effects of renal function remain unclear. The Relief for Acutely Fluid-Overloaded Patients With Decompensated Congestive Heart Failure (RAPID-CHF) trial randomized 40 individuals admitted with ADHF to ultrafiltration as initial therapy for 8 hours with progression to usual care versus usual care alone. The ultrafiltration group had more fluid removal after 24 and 48 hours than the usual care group (4650 mL vs 2838 mL, $P = .001$ at 24 hours, 8415 vs 5375 mL, $P = .012$ at 48 hours). Both groups experienced similar rises in SCr at the end of the 48-hour study period (+0.1 mg/dL).[44] The Ultrafiltration versus Intravenous Diuretics for Patients Hospitalized with Acute Decompensated Congestive Heart Failure (UNLOAD) trial found similar results. In the UNLOAD study, 200 individuals were randomized to ultrafiltration alone versus intravenous diuretics for 48 hours after enrollment (after 48 hours, the duration of ultrafiltration was determined by the treating physicians). Weight loss in the ultrafiltration group was greater at 48 hours 5.0 ± 3.1 kg versus 3.1 ± 3.5 kg, $P = .001$. Both groups once again had similar increases in SCr, with the proportion of individuals with an increase of at least 0.3 mg/dL similar in both groups (14.4% vs 7.7%, $P = .528$ at 24 hours, 26.5% vs 20.3%, $P = .430$ at 48 hours, 22.6% vs 19.8%, $P = .709$ at discharge). Further, there was no correlation between net fluid removal and changes in serum creatinine.[45] Although these studies suggest the increased benefit of additional fluid removal with ultrafiltration as compared with diuretics with no additional renal adverse effects, other studies have yet to confirm this benefit or demonstrate improvement in renal function with the use of ultrafiltration. A retrospective analysis of patients treated with ultrafiltration versus individuals treated with usual care alone or usual care with nesiritide found that those treated with ultrafiltration had higher rates of worsening renal function (SCr increase of at >0.5 mg/dL). Although patients treated with ultrafiltration were matched by age, renal function, ejection fraction, and etiology of heart failure with those receiving alternative regimens, the retrospective nature of the study makes it difficult to make definitive conclusions.[46] Thus, the role of ultrafiltration to prevent WRF in the setting of ADHF appears promising, but remains unclear.

Rather than focusing on the role of extracorporeal therapy and volume removal as a primary goal, other recent investigations have explored the role of adenosine in the setting of ADHF and its treatment. Tubuloglomerular feedback provides a mechanism to link distal sodium (and chloride) delivery to glomerular hemodynamics. Increased chloride delivery to the macula densa is sensed by the sodium-potassium-2-chloride cotransporter (NKCC2) and leads to the renal response of afferent arteriolar vasoconstriction, leading to decrease in single-nephron GFR. Knowing that adenosine, a mediator of the vasoconstriction reaction, acts via direct stimulation of adenosine receptor 1 (AR1) on the afferent arteriole has led to the investigation of AR1 receptor blockers on renal function in ADHF.[47] Givertz and colleagues[48] studied the effect of a novel A1 receptor antagonist, KW-3902, on diuresis and renal function in 2 groups of individuals: patients admitted with decompensated heart failure and renal dysfunction (estimated creatinine clearance between 20 mL/min and 80 mL/min) and patients admitted and currently treated for decompensated heart failure with treating physician–determined diuretic resistance. Individuals were randomized to 10 mg, 30 mg, or 60 mg of the study drug versus placebo in conjunction with intravenous furosemide. In the group of individuals with ADHF, 146 individuals received the study drug with a greater urine output in the first 6 hours, lower SCr at all dosages except the highest dose. Further, the treatment groups all had higher rates of premature treatment discontinuation because of goal diuresis achieved. At day 4, all the treatment groups had lower rates of WRF (defined by increase in serum creatinine >0.3 mg/dL) than the placebo group. However, the difference did not achieve statistical significance. In the diuretic-resistant protocol, 23 patients were treated with the A1 receptor antagonist and 12 individuals received placebo. At 6 and 24 hours, diuresis and natriuresis (urine output and urinary sodium excretion) were increased in the treatment group as compared with placebo. At

24 hours, the lowest and intermediate dose treatment arms were both associated with increased creatinine clearance as compared with the placebo and the highest dose group where creatinine clearance decreased. In both groups, rates of serious adverse events did not differ from placebo. An alternative A1 receptor antagonist, SLV 320, has also been studied with regard to its effects on both cardiac and renal function in the setting of congestive heart failure. A total of 111 individuals with NYHA Class II or III CHF, systolic dysfunction (EF <35%) and persistent edema were randomized to placebo, furosemide 40 mg or escalating doses of SLV 320 (5 mg intravenous [IV], 10 mg IV, or 15 mg IV). Individuals underwent pulmonary artery catheterization and had hemodynamic parameters followed throughout the study. After study drug infusion, urine volume, urinary sodium chloride, and potassium excretion as well as hemodynamic variables were compared among the 5 groups. Similar to the study of KW-3902, urine sodium and chloride excretion were greatest in the groups receiving the infusion of KW-3902 (at any dose) or furosemide. Urine volume was greater than placebo in the group of individuals receiving the 10-mg or 15-mg dose of KW-3902 as well as the group receiving furosemide. Importantly, the group of individuals receiving furosemide had a corresponding increase in serum cystatin-C, suggesting a fall in GFR. The groups of individuals receiving any dose of KW-3902 did not have a significant change in serum cystatin-C as compared with placebo, suggesting that the effect of increase sodium and water excretion occurred in the A1 receptor antagonist group without compromising renal function. However, the use of furosemide did have the effect of decreasing PCWP, whereas the use of the A1 receptor antagonist had no effect on PCWP.[49] It is unclear whether increasing the intensity of treatment with the A1 receptor antagonist to achieve a fall in PCWP, ie, a true therapeutic response, would also lead to a rise in serum cystatin C or evidence of WRF. Nevertheless, the study contributes to the increasing awareness of a potential novel and promising therapy of acute heart failure that preserves renal function. Although more investigation is required to define the optimal use of A1 receptor antagonists, the agents have a physiologic basis with initial human clinical data to suggest their effectiveness.

SUMMARY

Worsening renal function in the setting of congestive heart failure, both chronic and acute, is increasingly recognized as an independent predictor of poor prognosis. Further, it appears that small, even transient rises in SCr are clinically relevant. The introduction of urinary and serum biomarkers to identify kidney injury highlight the early stages where kidney injury occurs in the setting of heart failure, even before clinically apparent by increases in SCr. Further, the finding that biomarkers associated with renal tubular injury, as opposed to decreased filtration, are elevated in the setting of chronic and acute decompensated heart failure suggests "true" renal injury with heart failure and that optimization of cardiac function may not always be enough to restore renal function back to normal or reverse the damage that has occurred. The pathophysiology of worsening renal function in the setting of acute and chronic heart failure remains unclear, but different perspectives, focusing on venous congestion and intra-abdominal pressure, have offered alternative pathways to conventional thinking and serve as the stimulus for novel therapeutic interventions. Pharmacologic therapy has had minimal success in the past at improving renal outcomes; however, the novel agents offer some future promise. Extracorporeal therapy, although increasingly used and thought of as a treatment option, appears effective at increasing volume removal, but its effect on renal function remains varied. Future investigation directed at identifying which patients most benefit from each of these treatment strategies, along with the continued use of conventional ionotropes and vasodilators, is required to advance the treatment of the cardiorenal syndrome.

REFERENCES

1. Ronco C, House AA, Haapio M. Cardiorenal syndrome: refining the definition of a complex symbiosis gone wrong. Intensive Care Med 2008; 34(5):957–62.
2. Owan TE, Hodge DO, Herges RM, et al. Redfield. Secular trends in renal dysfunction and outcomes in hospitalized heart failure patients. J Card Fail 2006;12(4):257–62.
3. Smith GL, Lichtman JH, Bracken MB, et al. Renal impairment and outcomes in heart failure: systematic review and meta-analysis. J Am Coll Cardiol 2006;47:1987–96.
4. Jessup M, Costanzo MR. The cardiorenal syndrome: do we need a change of strategy or a change of tactics? J Am Coll Cardiol 2009;53:597–9.
5. Al-Ahmad A, Rand WM, Manjunath G, et al. Reduced kidney function and anemia as risk factors for mortality in patients with left ventricular dysfunction. J Am Coll Cardiol 2001;38:955–62.
6. Khan NA, Ma I, Thompson CR, et al. Kidney function and mortality among patients with left ventricular systolic dysfunction. J Am Soc Nephrol 2006;17: 244–53.
7. Weiner DE, Krassilnikova M, Hocine T, et al. CKD classification based on estimated GFR over three years and subsequent cardiac and mortality outcomes: a cohort study. BMC Nephrol 2009;10: 26–37.
8. Tsutsui H, Tsuchihashi-Makaya M, Kinugawa S, et al. Clinical characteristics and outcome of hospitalized patients with heart failure in Japan: Rationale and Design of Japanese Cardiac Registry of Heart Failure in Cardiology (JCARE-CARD). Circ J 2006; 70:1617–23.
9. Cowie MR, Komajda M, Murray-Thomas T, et al. Prevalence and impact of worsening renal function in patients hospitalized with decompensated heart failure: results of the prospective outcomes study in heart failure. Eur Heart J 2006;27:1216–22.
10. Metra M, Nodari S, Parrinello G, et al. Worsening renal function in patients hospitalized for acute heart failure: clinical implications and prognostic significance. Eur J Heart Fail 2008;10(2):188–95.
11. Logeart D, Tabet JY, Hittinger L, et al. Transient worsening of renal function during hospitalization for acute heart failure alters outcome. Int J Cardiol 2008;127(2):228–32.
12. Weisbord SD, Chen H, Stone RA, et al. Associations of increases in serum creatinine with mortality and length of hospital stay after coronary angiography. J Am Soc Nephrol 2006;17(10):2871–7.
13. Lassnigg A, Schmidlin D, Mouhieddine M, et al. Minimal changes of serum creatinine predict prognosis in patients after cardiothoracic surgery: a prospective cohort study. J Am Soc Nephrol 2004;15:1597–605.
14. Joannidis M, Metnitz B, Bauer P, et al. Acute kidney injury in critically ill patients classified by AKIN versus RIFLE using the SAPS 3 database. Intensive Care Med 2009;35(10):1692–702.
15. Bagshaw SM, George C, Bellomo R, et al. A comparison of the RIFLE and AKIN criteria for acute kidney injury in critically ill patients. Nephrol Dial Transplant. 2008;23(5):1569–74.
16. Mullens W, Abrahams Z, Francis GS, et al. Importance of venous congestion for worsening of renal function in advanced decompensated heart failure. J Am Coll Cardiol 2009;53:589–96.
17. Nohria A, Hasselblad V, Stebbins A, et al. Cardiorenal interactions: insights from the ESCAPE trial. J Am Coll Cardiol 2008;51:1268–74.
18. Damman K, Navis G, Smilde TD, et al. Decreased cardiac output, venous congestion and the association with renal impairment in patients with cardiac dysfunction. Eur J Heart Fail 2007;9: 872–8.

19. Wathen RL, Selkurt EE. Intrarenal regulatory factors of salt excretion during renal venous pressure elevation. Am J Physiol 1969;216:1517–24.

20. Burnett JC, Knox FG. Renal interstitial pressure and sodium excretion during renal vein constriction. Am J Physiol 1980;238:F279–82.

21. Dalfino L, Tullo L, Donadio I, et al. Intra-abdominal hypertension and acute renal failure in critically ill patients. Intensive Care Med 2008;34:707–13.

22. Regueira T, Bruhn A, Hasbun P, et al. Intra-abdominal hypertension: incidence and association with organ dysfunction during early septic shock. J Crit Care 2008;23(4):461–7.

23. Mullens W, Abrahams Z, Skouri HN, et al. Elevated intrabdominal pressure in acute decompensated heart failure. J Am Coll Cardiol 2008;51:300–6.

24. Mullens W, Abrahams Z, Francis GS, et al. Prompt reduction in intra-abdominal pressure following large-volume mechanical fluid removal improves renal insufficiency in refractory decompensated heart failure. J Cardiac Fail 2008;14:508–14.

25. Van De Wal RM, Asselbergs FW, Plokker HW, et al. High prevalence of microalbuminuria in chronic heart failure patients. J Card Fail 2005;11:602–6.

26. Bonventre JV. Diagnosis of acute kidney injury: from classic parameters to new biomarkers. Contrib Nephrol 2007;156:213–9.

27. Nickolas T, Barasch J, Devarajan P. Biomarkers in acute and chronic kidney disease. Curr Opin Nephrol Hypertens 2008;17:127–32.

28. Poniatowski B, Malyzsko J, Bachorzewska-Gajewska H, et al. Serum neutrophil gelatinase-associated lipocalin as a marker of renal function in patients with chronic heart failure and coronary artery disease. Kidney Blood Press Res 2009;32:77–80.

29. Yndestad A, Landrø L, Ueland T, et al. Increased systemic and myocardial expression of neutrophil gelatinase-associated lipocalin in clinical and experimental heart failure. Eur Heart J 2009;10:1229–36.

30. Garg R, Yusuf F. Overview of randomized trials of angiotensin-converting enzyme inhibitors on mortality and morbidity in patients with heart failure: Collaborative Group on ACE Inhibitor Trials. JAMA 1995;273(18):1450–6.

31. Flather MD, Yusuf S, Kober L, et al. Long-term ACE-inhibitor therapy in patients with heart failure or left-ventricular dysfunction: a systematic overview of data from individual patients. ACE-Inhibitor Myocardial Infoarction Collaborative Group. Lancet 2000; 355(9215):1575–81.

32. Pfeffer MA, Swedberg K, Granger CB, et al. Effects of candesartan on mortality and morbidity in patients with chronic heart failure: the CHARM-Overall programme. Lancet 2003;362:759–66.

33. Masoudi FA, Rathore SS, Wang Y, et al. National patterns of use and effectiveness of angiotensin converting enzyme inhibitors in older patients with heart failure and left ventricular systolic dysfunction. Circulation 2004;110:724–31.

34. deGroote P, Isnard R, Assyag P, et al. Is the gap between guidelines and clinical practice in heart failure treatment being filled? Insights from the IMPACT RECO survey. Eur J Heart Fail 2007;12: 1205–11.

35. Manyemba J, Mangoni AA, Pettingale KW, et al. Determinants of failure to prescribe target doses of angiotensin-converting enzyme inhibitors for heart failure. Eur J Heart Fail 2003;5:693–6.

36. Ahmed A, Love TE, Sui X, et al. Effects of angiotensin-converting enzyme inhibitors in systolic heart failure patients with chronic kidney disease. J Cardiac Fail 2006;12:499–506.

37. Anand IS, Bishu K, Rector TS, et al. Proteinuria, chronic kidney disease, and the effect of an angiotensin receptor blocker in addition to an angiotensin-converting enzyme inhibitor in patients with moderate to severe heart failure. Circulation 2009; 120:1577–84.

38. Bakris GL, Weir M. Angiotensin converting enzyme inhibitor associated elevations in serum creatinine: is this a cause for concern? Arch Intern Med 2000; 160:685–93.

39. McMurray JJ, Pitt B, Latini R, et al. Effects of the oral direct renin inhibitor aliskiren in patients with symptomatic heart failure. Circ Heart Fail 2008;1:17–24.

40. Pitt B, Zannad F, Remme WJ, et al. The effects of spironolactone on morbidity and mortality in patients with severe heart failure: Randomized Aldactone Evaluation Study Investigators. N Engl J Med 1999;341:709–17.

41. Pitt B, Remme WJ, Zannad F, et al. Eplerenone, a selective aldosterone blocker in patients with left ventricular dysfunction after myocardial infarction. N Engl J Med 2003;348:1309–21.

42. Juurlink DN, Mamdani MM, Lee DS, et al. Rates of hyperkalemia after publication of the Randomized Aldactone Evaluation Study. N Engl J Med 2004; 351:543–51.

43. Edwards NC, Steeds RP, Stewart PM, et al. Effect of spironolactone on left ventricular mass and aortic stiffness in early-stage chronic kidney disease. J Am Coll Cardiol 2009;54:505–12.

44. Bart BA, Boyle A, Bank AJ, et al. Ultrafiltration versus usual care for hospitalized patients with heart failure. The Relief for Acutely Fluid-Overloaded Patients with Decompensated Congestive Heart Failure (RAPID-CHF) Trial. J Am Coll Cardiol 2005;46:2043–6.

45. Constanzo MR, Guglin ME, Saltzberg MT, et al. Ultrafiltration versus intravenous diuretics for patients hospitalized for acute decompensated heart failure. J Am Coll Cardiol 2007;49:675–83.

46. Bartone C, Saghir S, Menon SG, et al. Comparison of ultrafiltration, nesiritide, and usual care in acute

decompensated heart failure. Congest Heart Fail 2008;14:298–301.

47. Sun D, Samuelson LC, Yang T, et al. Mediation of tubuloglomerular feedback by adenosine: evidence form mice lacking adenosine 1 receptors. Proc Natl Acad Sci U S A 2001;14:9983–8.

48. Givertz MM, Massie BM, Fields TK, et al. The effects of KW-3902, an adenosine A1-receptor antagonist, on diuresis and renal function in patients with acute decompensated heart failure and renal impairment or diuretic resistance. J Am Coll Cardiol 2007;50: 1551–60.

49. Mitrovic V, Seferovic P, Dodic S, et al. Cardio-renal effects of the A1 adenosine receptor antagonist SLV320 in patients with heart failure. Circ Heart Fail 2009;2:523–31.

Diabetes, Cardiovascular Risk and Nephropathy

Allison J. Hahr, MD, Mark E. Molitch, MD*

KEYWORDS

- Diabetes mellitus • Cardiovascular risk
- Nephropathy • Risk reduction

Approximately 7% of the population of the United States has diabetes mellitus (DM), which represents nearly 24 million adults and children, and about 250 million people worldwide are affected by type 2 diabetes. The incidence continues to increase, likely because of the increase in obesity and age of the population. Diabetes-related deaths represented about 5% of all deaths in 2000.[1] Diabetes is well known to be associated with multiple complications that contribute to its significant morbidity and mortality. The microvascular complications, including retinopathy and nephropathy, are widely recognized, as are the macrovascular complications. Of the associated macrovascular complications, cardiovascular disease (CVD) is the major contributor representing the largest cause of morbidity and mortality and related costs of diabetes care.[2] CVD is the leading cause of death among individuals with diabetes, accounting for about 65% of all deaths.[3] A relationship between diabetes and CVD has been clearly established and is discussed in detail in this article.

CVD IN DIABETES
High Prevalence of CVD in Diabetes

Individuals with diabetes have high rates of CVD. Cohorts from the Framingham Heart Study who were at least 50 years old and had no evidence of CVD at baseline were followed to assess their lifetime risk of developing CVD. Increased cholesterol and blood pressure were associated with increased risk of CVD. Diabetes represented the largest single risk factor, with 57.3% of women and 67.1% of men with diabetes developing CVD compared with 16.3% and 30.2% of age-matched women and men without diabetes.[4] In a study of participants drawn from the Framingham Heart Study, the lifetime risk of CVD was assessed in patients with and without diabetes and stratified by obesity. At 30 years of follow-up, 67.1% of women with diabetes had developed CVD compared with 38% of women without diabetes. Similarly, 78% of men with diabetes were affected compared with 54.8% of men without diabetes. The lifetime risk of CVD further increased with weight.[5] Individuals with type 2 diabetes carry an increased risk of CVD even before clinical diagnosis, perhaps in part related to coexisting risk factors and delayed diagnosis. Nearly 120,000 women in the Nurses' Health Study were followed for 20 years and assessed for diabetes during the course of the study. Of women who were newly diagnosed with type 2 diabetes, the relative risk of myocardial infarction (MI) was 3.17 compared with women who never developed diabetes, suggesting that it would be beneficial to identify individuals at risk for diabetes and intensively treat associated risk factors even before they meet criteria diagnostic of diabetes.[6]

Mortality of CVD in Diabetes

More individuals with diabetes experience cardiovascular (CV)-related deaths than individuals without diabetes. In a study of Australian patients,

Division of Endocrinology, Metabolism, and Molecular Medicine, Northwestern University Feinberg School of Medicine, 645 North Michigan Avenue, Suite 530, Chicago, IL 60611, USA
* Corresponding author.
E-mail address: molitch@northwestern.edu

Cardiol Clin 28 (2010) 467–475
doi:10.1016/j.ccl.2010.04.006

subjects were observed for 4 weeks after presenting to the hospital with their first MI. Men and women with established diabetes had a relative risk of death of 1.25 and 1.56 compared with men and women without diabetes.[7] In a study looking at long-term survival, nearly 2000 patients hospitalized with an MI were then followed for nearly 4 years after presenting to a medical center in the United States. Individuals with diabetes had a higher overall mortality compared with those without diabetes, with an adjusted hazard ratio (HR) of 1.7, and this risk was even higher in women.[8] In a meta-analysis of prospective cohort studies conducted by Huxley and colleagues[9] of coronary heart disease (CHD) in men and women with and without type 2 diabetes, 5.4% of those with diabetes died of CHD compared with 1.6% of those without diabetes. Data from a subset analysis of the Thrombolysis in Myocardial Infarction (TIMI) Study Group following patients 1 month and 1 year after presenting with acute coronary syndromes showed consistently higher mortality at both time points in patients with diabetes compared with those without.[10] Women in the Nurses' Health Study were followed for 20 years, and those with diabetes and CHD had a relative risk of death of 6.84 compared with age-matched women with neither condition; the relative risk of fatal CHD was 25.8.[11] A study of deaths related to diabetes showed an improvement in rates of death among men with diabetes from 1971 to 2000, but not among women.[12] Comparing women with and without diabetes, the difference in all-cause mortality increased more than twofold in the same period.[12]

Diabetes as a CVD Risk Equivalent

Multiple studies have shown diabetes as a risk equivalent to coronary artery disease and previous MI. Haffner and colleagues[13] followed patients for 7 years, finding that patients with diabetes with no previous history of MI carried as high a risk of death as patients without diabetes but a known history of MI. In a prospective study in Scotland following subjects for 25 years, the HR for vascular mortality for individuals only affected by diabetes compared with those with only known CVD was 1.97 and 1.17 for women and men, respectively, indicating that the risk of vascular death is as high in those with diabetes as in those with CVD alone, if not higher.[14] Similarly, in a population-based study in Finland, men and women with diabetes without a previous MI had comparable rates of death with those with a previous MI but no diabetes.[15] Furthermore, individuals with diabetes and no evidence of any type of CHD had an even

higher risk of death compared with subjects with known CHD but no diabetes.[15] A large study in Demark of individuals aged 30 years and older showed that CV risk was similar in those with diabetes who had no known CVD to those without diabetes with a previous history of MI. The HR for CV death for men with diabetes and without was 2.42 and 2.44; for women, the HR was 2.45 and 2.62, and the type of diabetes did not alter the results.[16]

These studies show that individuals with diabetes carry as high a risk of MI and CVD as those with known CVD. Thus, an individual with diabetes needs aggressive measures for prevention of CVD and control of its risk factors. Diabetes as a risk equivalent has led to the establishment of guidelines to treat it as such. The Adult Treatment Panel III report of the National Cholesterol Education Program considers patients with diabetes without CHD to be of similar risk to individuals with known CHD, and thus suggests similar lipid management guidelines for the 2 groups.[17]

RISK FACTORS FOR CVD IN DIABETES

As noted, individuals with diabetes have high rates of CVD. This can be partly explained by the high prevalence of coexisting diseases such as nephropathy, dyslipidemias, hypertension, and obesity. This article provides a brief summary (see the articles by Polonsky and Locatelli, Hopkins and Bakris, Saha and Tuttle, and Sorrentino elsewhere in this issue for further exploration of these topics).

Nephropathy

As discussed earlier, diabetes is a strong risk factor for CVD and is considered the equivalent of such. CVD is the leading cause of death in patients with stage 5 chronic kidney disease (CKD).[18,19] Thus, the combination of the two is particularly robust in terms of CVD risk. When patients with stage 5 CKD are divided into those with and without diabetes, the annual mortality is increased by about 40% in those with diabetes.[20,21] Conversely, when individuals with type 1 and type 2 diabetes are divided into those with and without evidence of CKD, the CVD risk is higher in those with evidence of diabetic kidney disease, even at the early stage of microalbuminuria (30–300 mg/g creatinine),[18–19,22–24] and the risk increases as the kidney disease progresses to clinical albuminuria (>300 mg/g creatinine) and then decreased glomerular filtration rate (GFR).[20,22] Thus, control of CVD risk factors is particularly important in any individual who has diabetes, CKD, and particularly both. There are many risk factors for CVD in people with diabetes and CKD, including dyslipidemias, hypertension, obesity, and hyperglycemia, and intensive management should be pursued.[21,25,26]

Diabetic Dyslipidemias

Dyslipidemias are a major risk factor for CVD in populations with and without diabetes.[17,27] Type 1 diabetes is usually associated with normal low-density lipoprotein (LDL) and high-density lipoprotein (HDL) cholesterol levels and increased triglyceride levels, the latter being due primarily to poor glycemic control.[27,28] Poor control with inadequate insulin leads to a reduction in the activity of lipoprotein lipase and consequent inability to clear chylomicrons and very low-density lipoprotein (VLDL).[28,29] When control is poor, HDL cholesterol levels may also be decreased and LDL cholesterol levels increased.[27] Type 2 diabetes is generally associated with reduced HDL cholesterol levels, increased triglyceride levels, and normal LDL cholesterol levels, although there is a shift in the LDL particle size to the more atherogenic small, dense LDL particles.[28] The reduction of HDL cholesterol is due primarily to an increased transfer of cholesterol from HDL to triglyceride-rich lipoproteins with concomitant transfer of triglycerides to HDL. These triglyceride-rich particles are then hydrolyzed by hepatic lipase and rapidly catabolized and cleared.[28] Insulin resistance increases hepatic lipase activity, which then hydrolyzes phospholipids in LDL and HDL particles, leading to smaller, denser LDL particles and a decrease in the HDL_2 subspecies.[28]

The reduction of LDL levels using statins has proved to be beneficial for patients with normal kidney function with and without diabetes with respect to the risk for CVD. Based on the results of multiple trials showing efficacy at lower starting and target LDL cholesterol levels (Heart Protection Study, Collaborative Atorvastatin Diabetes Study [CARDS], the Pravastatin or Atorvastatin Evaluation and Infection Therapy-Thrombolysis in Myocardial Infarction [PROVE-IT] and the Treat to New Targets [TNT] studies[29–33]), the Adult Treatment Panel III of the National Cholesterol Education Program in 2004 issued a modification of their 2002 Guidelines, indicating that in patients at very high risk, an LDL cholesterol goal of less than 70 mg/dL, even in those starting with levels less than 100 mg/dL, is a reasonable therapeutic option.[34] Treatment with statins should be considered irrespective of baseline lipid levels given the high CVD risk associated with CKD in diabetes. On average, fasting lipid levels should be obtained annually in patients with diabetes.[2] In those with increased lipids, lifestyle management focusing on weight reduction, augmenting activity, and improving diet is advised. In general, in addition to controlling LDL, efforts should be made to achieve goal triglyceride levels of less than 150 mg, and goal HDL cholesterol of more than 40 mg/dL in men and more than 50 mg/dL in women.

Whether statins should be used in diabetic and other patients with impaired GFRs is not well established, because patients with impaired GFR were usually excluded from the statin trials. However, post-hoc analyses of diabetic and nondiabetic individuals with stage 3 CKD who were included in these trials generally show benefit of lowering LDL levels with statins on CVD outcomes.[35] However, 2 prospective, randomized studies have shown no benefit of statin use on CVD outcomes in patients on dialysis with and without diabetes.[36,37] It is not clear why benefit does not extend to these patients, but it may be that the CVD in such patients is so far advanced that LDL lowering with statins is no longer efficacious.

Blood Pressure Control

Hypertension is commonly seen in patients with diabetes and is a major risk factor in the development of microvascular disease and CVD. In type 1 diabetes, hypertension is usually a consequence of nephropathy, whereas in type 2 diabetes hypertension may be present independent of nephropathy. Increased blood pressure is associated with progression of CKD as well as CVD in diabetes, and optimizing blood pressure control is important in decreasing the progression of nephropathy.[38] Several studies have shown the association between progression of nephropathy and increase in blood pressure.[39–41] Blood pressure should be checked at every office visit, with hypertension defined as a systolic blood pressure greater than or equal to 130 mm Hg or diastolic blood pressure greater than or equal to 80 mm Hg on 2 separate readings for anyone with diabetes or CKD.[42] Goal blood pressure in diabetes is a systolic blood pressure less than 130 mm Hg and diastolic blood pressure less than 80 mm Hg.[43] Selective additional benefits of drugs active in blockade of the renin-angiotensin-aldosterone system are discussed in the articles by Hopkins and Bakris, and Calhoun and Sharma elsewhere in this issue.

Nutrition and Weight Control

Lifestyle modification is an integral part of diabetes management. Management of nutrition in a patient with diabetes can be complex but necessary, with the focus on weight management, reduction in unhealthy fat and cholesterol intake, and attainment of glucose control. For diabetes in general, weight loss can reduce insulin resistance, thus a goal body mass index (BMI) of less than 25 kg/m^2 is desirable. This BMI can be achieved by the use of low-calorie carbohydrate or fat-restricted diets. In either diet, it is important to restrict saturated fat and trans fats, given the effect on dyslipidemia. Carbohydrate intake needs to be assessed in any individual with diabetes and followed closely.[2] In those with CKD, other aspects of diet, such as salt, potassium, and protein, are important and are dealt in the articles by Polonsky and Locatelli, Whaley-Connell and Kalaitzidis, Hopkins and Bakris, and Sorrentino elsewhere in this issue.[38]

CVD AND GLUCOSE INCREASES

The incidence of complications related to diabetes increases with higher levels of hyperglycemia, and this relationship is also noted with CVD. In a meta-analysis of observational studies of the relationship between hemoglobin A1c (HbA1c) and CVD, an 18% increased risk of CVD was seen for every 1% increase in HbA1c.[44] In the Heart Outcome Prevention Evaluation (HOPE) study, a 1% increase in HbA1c was linked to higher rates of nephropathy (rate ratio [RR] 1.34, $P<.0001$), CV events (RR 1.07, $P = .014$) and death (RR 1.12, $P = .0004$).[45] Hyperglycemia is also linked to higher rates of CVD. Selvin and colleagues[46] studied the relationship between HbA1c and CVD and found that higher levels of HbA1c conferred an increased risk of CVD, even in individuals without diabetes.

The increased rate of CV events in diabetes may be explained by the presence of multiple additional CV risk factors, including dyslipidemia, hypertension, nephropathy, and obesity. However, there is a suggestion that the way glycemic control is achieved also matters. Many studies suggest that postprandial (PP) glucose increases contribute to the development of CV complications more than fasting blood glucose (FBG) levels and regardless of HbA1c, thereby making PP glucose levels an ideal target for intervention to reduce diabetes-related morbidity and mortality. Postprandial hyperglycemia has been implicated as causing vascular endothelial damage by means of oxidative stress and contributing to atherosclerosis, an observation made independently of the effects of PP hyperlipidemia.[47] The isolated increase of PP glucose with normal FBGs levels is common. Thus, not everyone with diabetes is diagnosed based on a screening fasting glucose, necessitating use of the 2 hour oral glucose tolerance test (OGTT) for the diagnosis of diabetes. In the Diabetes

Epidemiology: Collaborative Analysis Of Diagnostic Criteria in Europe (DECODE) study, high 2-hour PP glucose levels led to increased risk of death from all causes and CVD, independent of FBG.[48] The Hoorn study showed that 2-hour PP glucose levels were better predictors of increased death rates from CVD compared with HbA1c.[49] An analysis of data from National Health and Nutrition Examination Survey II (NHANES II) participants showed that adults with PP glucose increases greater than or equal to 200 mg/dL but normal fasting glucose levels (<126 mg/dL) had a relative hazard of 1.4 for CVD-related deaths compared with those with normal fasting and PP glucoses.[49] The HEART2D trial studied CV outcomes in patients with type 2 diabetes after an acute MI who were treated with basal insulin or prandial insulin only. HbA1c levels were similar between the 2 groups, and there was no observed difference in CV events despite differences in fasting and PP blood glucoses.[50]

GLYCEMIC CONTROL AND INFLUENCE ON CVD
Type 1 Diabetes

There have been multiple interventional studies of the association between tight glycemic control and CVD. The Diabetes Control and Complications Trial (DCCT) was a multicenter, randomized, clinical trial of 1441 subjects with type 1 diabetes that compared the effects of intensive diabetes treatment with conventional diabetes treatment on the development and progression of the long-term complications of type 1 diabetes. Subjects were followed for a mean of 6.5 years. At baseline, mean HbA1clevels were similar in both treatment groups. By 3 months after randomization, mean HbA1c was approximately 2% lower in the intensive treatment group than in the conventional treatment group, and this difference was maintained throughout the study (7.2% vs 9.1%, $P<.001$).[51] The intensive treatment group experienced significantly less microvascular disease, including retinopathy, nephropathy, and neuropathy.

To assess the effect on progression of microvascular disease, neuropathic disease, and CVD, 1349 of these DCCT subjects were then followed in the Epidemiology of Diabetes Interventions and Complications (EDIC) study for several more years. Subjects were returned to the care of their own physicians and were no longer maintained in different treatment groups. The previous difference in HbA1c for the intensive versus the conventional group in the DCCT gradually narrowed in the first 2 years of the follow-up period and then remained near 8% for both groups in the subsequent years. Subjects were evaluated for progression of microvascular and neurologic complications as well as the onset of any CVD-related event, which included death, MI (nonfatal or subclinical), stroke, angina, ischemia, and need for revascularization.[52] In the DCCT, the intensive treatment group had lower rates of microalbuminuria and albuminuria and lower HbA1c values, which likely relates to lower CV risk. Long-term follow-up in EDIC showed the persistence of the beneficial effects of this previous intensive glycemic control because this treatment group maintained lower rates of microalbuminuria despite an increase in HbA1c to that of the conventional treatment group. Other CVD parameters, such as blood pressure and lipids, were not significantly different between the 2 groups.

In the DCCT, the intensive glycemic control group had fewer CV events, but the difference was not significant. This result was believed to be due in part to the younger age of the subjects and low number of events.[51] In the time period encompassing both studies, a mean of 17 years of previous intensive treatment reduced the time to a first CV event by 42% compared with conventional treatment. In addition, risk of death, nonfatal MI, or stroke was reduced by 57% in those with intensive glycemic control. Presence of microalbuminuria or albuminuria further increased the risk of CVD in the conventional treatment group, and the difference in CV disease risk between the 2 groups continued to be significant after adjustment for the presence of kidney disease.[52]

Type 2 Diabetes

Multiple trials have shown the beneficial effects of tight glycemic control on microvascular complications in type 2 diabetes; however, the effect on macrovascular disease has been less clear. A similar result to the DCCT/EDIC was noted in the United Kingdom Prospective Diabetes Study (UKPDS) in which patients with newly diagnosed type 2 diabetes were randomly assigned to intensive management using a sulfonylurea or insulin, or to conventional treatment with diet alone. The average HbA1c for the intensive group was 7.0% compared with 7.9% for the conventional group during the study. Microvascular disease was significantly reduced by 25% in the intensive treatment group (P = .0099), but not macrovascular disease, with a reduction in the risk of MI and sudden death of 16% observed but not significant (P = .052).[53] Subjects from the UKPDS were then followed for up to 10 years, at which point they no longer continued to have differences in glucose control

and maintained similar HbA1c levels starting about 1 year after follow-up. In this subsequent study, the previous intensive treatment group had a 15% reduction in MI (P = .01) and 13% reduction in death from all causes (P = .007), indicating a benefit of tight long-term glycemic control.[54]

A subset of patients from the UKPDS who were overweight (>120% of their ideal body weight) were randomized to intensive treatment with a sulfonylurea or insulin, conventional treatment with diet alone or treatment with metformin. Those treated with metformin had a reduction in death from any cause of 36% (P = .011) and reduction in MI of 39% (P = .01) compared with those treated with diet alone.[55] In the follow-up study, reductions in CVD continued to be observed, including a 33% decreased risk of MI (P = .005) and a 27% reduction in death from any cause (P = .002).[54]

In the Steno-2 study, the effect of tight glycemic, blood pressure, and cholesterol control in 160 patients with type 2 diabetes and established microalbuminuria on microvascular disease, CVD, and mortality was assessed.[56,57] Patients in the intensive group had an HbA1c of 7.9% compared with 9% in those in the conventional treatment group. In the initial study of nearly 8 years' duration, those with intensive treatment had lower rates of nephropathy (HR, 0.39; P = .003) and CVD (HR, 0.47; P = .01).[56] In the subsequent follow-up study that lasted more than 5 years, the subjects were given information regarding the benefits of glycemic control and returned to the care of community diabetes specialists. During the entire study totaling more than 13 years, members of the intensive treatment group had lower rates of CV events (HR, 0.41; P<.001) and CV-related deaths (HR, 0.43; P = .04). Death from any cause was also significantly reduced (HR, 0.54; P = .02).[57] How much of the benefit in this study can be attributed to glycemic control versus blood pressure and cholesterol control cannot be determined exactly. Nevertheless, the investigators used a risk calculator and found that the use of blood pressure control agents and statins may have had the largest effect, followed by the use of diabetic therapies and aspirin.[57]

In the Action in Diabetes and Vascular disease: Preterax and Diamicron Modified Release Controlled Evaluation (ADVANCE) trial, 11,140 subjects with type 2 diabetes were randomized to intensive control with gliclazide and additional therapy (HbA1c 6.5%) or standard control (HbA1c 7.3%; P<.001) and followed for approximately 5 years. The study was designed to follow microvascular and macrovascular events. Those receiving intensive therapy had a significant reduction in new-onset microalbuminuria (HR,

0.91; $P = .02$). However, intensive control did not reduce the number of macrovascular events (HR, 0.94; $P = .32$), CV-related deaths (HR, 0.88; $P = .12$), or deaths from any cause (HR, 0.93; $P = .28$). A higher rate of hypoglycemia was observed in the intensive treatment group.[58]

The Action to Control Cardiovascular Risk in Diabetes Study Group (ACCORD) also studied CV events in patients with type 2 diabetes. Subjects had a baseline HbA1c greater than 7.5% and had previously established CVD or CVD risk factors. During the study, there were increased risks of hypoglycemia and weight gain in the group assigned to an HbA1c target of less than 6.0% (and achieving an HbA1c of 6.4%) compared with the group assigned to an HbA1c target of 7.0% to 7.9% (and achieving a target of 7.5%). There was no significant difference in CV events; however, deaths from all causes were more frequent in the intensive group, (HR, 1.22; $P = .04$), leading to early termination of the study. The increased mortality risk could not be attributed specifically to hypoglycemia.[59]

The Veterans Affairs Diabetes Trial (VADT) also studied risk of CV events in patients with type 2 diabetes: 1791 veterans with type 2 diabetes and a baseline HbA1c of greater than 7.5% were randomized to intensive or conventional treatment. The average age of subjects was 60.4 years, with mean time since diagnosis of diabetes of 11.5 years. Nearly half of the subjects already had known CVD. After follow-up for 5 to 8 years, the intensive therapy group achieved an HbA1c of 6.9% compared with 8.4% in the conventional treatment group. Subjects were followed for time to first CV event, and no significant difference in rates was found between the 2 groups. In addition, no difference in the rate of death from any cause or microvascular complications was seen.[60] Therefore, these recent data from ADVANCE, ACCORD, and VADT have not shown a benefit of achieving HbA1c levels of less than 7.0% in reducing CV outcomes in individuals with established type 2 diabetes. Large differences in HbA1c levels between the intensive and conventional treatment group were not attained in the studies, and thus it should not be assumed that any level of glycemic control would impart benefit toward reduction of CVD.[61] Additional CV risk factors were treated in the studies, which may have affected the CVD event rates.[61]

Insulin resistance has long been postulated to have an important role in the pathogenesis of increased CVD risk in patients with type 2 diabetes,[62] with the implication that treatments of diabetes that would reduce insulin resistance might have a specific effect on CVD. This hypothesis was directly tested by the Bypass Angioplasty Revascularization Investigation 2 Diabetes (BARI 2D) study, which found no significant difference in CVD outcomes when diabetes treatment was directed at reducing insulin resistance versus providing increased insulin.[63] However, those with the most advanced coronary artery disease, as documented by coronary angiography, seemed to benefit from treatment directed at reducing insulin resistance.[63]

Glycemic control is important for CVD risk reduction, but these recent studies do not support an HbA1c target of less than 7.0%. Although there may be a subset of individuals with advanced coronary artery disease (that can only be diagnosed by angiography) who benefit from treatments directed at the reduction of insulin resistance, in general the focus should be on improvement in glycemic control rather than the use of specific classes of medications.

SUMMARY

Diabetic patients with CKD are at extraordinarily high risk for CVD, and the greater the amount of CKD, the greater the risk. Therefore, all aspects of risk reduction should be rigorously applied to such patients. Statins should be used with reduction of LDL cholesterol levels to less than 70 mg/dL in all such patients. Although no benefit of such reduction has been shown in patients with diabetes on dialysis, it is not known whether statins should be withdrawn when patients start on dialysis. Blood pressure management is also important, with a goal of less than 130/80 mm Hg and perhaps even lower. Although glycemic control may be less important than the reduction of other risk factors for CVD outcomes, it nonetheless remains critically important for reduction in the development and progression of retinopathy, neuropathy, and even nephropathy itself. Other risk factor reduction, such as smoking cessation and weight reduction, should also be implemented. As the Steno-2 study showed, multiple risk factor reduction can have a large effect on reduction of CVD outcomes.

REFERENCES

1. Roglic G, Unwin N, Bennett PH, et al. The burden of mortality attributable to diabetes: realistic estimates for the year 2000. Diabetes Care 2005;28(9):2130–5.
2. American Diabetes Association. Standards of Medical Care in Diabetes—2010. Diabetes Care 2010;33(Suppl 1):S11–61.
3. Thom T, Haase N, Rosamond W, et al. Heart disease and stroke statistics–2006 update: a report from the

American Heart Association Statistics Committee and Stroke Statistics Subcommittee. Circulation 2006;113(6):e85–151.

4. Lloyd-Jones DM, Leip EP, Larson MG, et al. Prediction of lifetime risk for cardiovascular disease by risk factor burden at 50 years of age. Circulation 2006; 113(6):791–8.

5. Fox CS, Pencina MJ, Wilson PW, et al. Lifetime risk of cardiovascular disease among individuals with and without diabetes stratified by obesity status in the Framingham heart study. Diabetes Care 2008; 31(8):1582–4.

6. Hu FB, Stampfer MJ, Haffner SM, et al. Elevated risk of cardiovascular disease before clinical diagnosis of type 2 diabetes. Diabetes Care 2002;25(7):1129–34.

7. Chun BY, Dobson AJ, Heller RF. The impact of diabetes on survival among patients with first myocardial infarction. Diabetes Care 1997;20(5): 704–8.

8. Mukamal KJ, Nesto RW, Cohen MC, et al. Impact of diabetes on long-term survival after acute myocardial infarction: comparability of risk with prior myocardial infarction. Diabetes Care 2001;24(8):1422–7.

9. Huxley R, Barzi F, Woodward M. Excess risk of fatal coronary heart disease associated with diabetes in men and women: meta-analysis of 37 prospective cohort studies. BMJ 2006;332(7533):73–8.

10. Donahoe SM, Stewart GC, McCabe CH, et al. Diabetes and mortality following acute coronary syndromes. JAMA 2007;298(7):765–75.

11. Hu FB, Stampfer MJ, Solomon CG, et al. The impact of diabetes mellitus on mortality from all causes and coronary heart disease in women: 20 years of follow-up. Arch Intern Med 2001;161(14): 1717–23.

12. Gregg EW, Gu Q, Cheng YJ, et al. Mortality trends in men and women with diabetes, 1971 to 2000. Ann Intern Med 2007;147(3):149–55.

13. Haffner SM, Lehto S, Ronnemaa T, et al. Mortality from coronary heart disease in subjects with type 2 diabetes and in nondiabetic subjects with and without prior myocardial infarction. N Engl J Med 1998;339(4):229–34.

14. Whiteley L, Padmanabhan S, Hole D, et al. Should diabetes be considered a coronary heart disease risk equivalent? results from 25 years of follow-up in the Renfrew and Paisley survey. Diabetes Care 2005;28(7):1588–93.

15. Juutilainen A, Lehto S, Ronnemaa T, et al. Type 2 diabetes as a "coronary heart disease equivalent": an 18-year prospective population-based study in Finnish subjects. Diabetes Care 2005; 28(12):2901–7.

16. Schramm TK, Gislason GH, Kober L, et al. Diabetes patients requiring glucose-lowering therapy and nondiabetics with a prior myocardial infarction carry the same cardiovascular risk: a population study of 3.3 million people. Circulation 2008; 117(15):1945–54.

17. Expert Panel on Detection, Evaluation, And Treatment of High Blood Cholesterol In Adults. Executive Summary of the Third Report of the National Cholesterol Education Program (NCEP) Expert Panel on Detection, Evaluation, and Treatment of High Blood Cholesterol in Adults (Adult Treatment Panel III). JAMA 2001;285(19):2486–97.

18. Jensen T, Borch-Johnsen K, Kofoed-Enevoldsen A, et al. Coronary heart disease in young type 1 (insulin-dependent) diabetic patients with and without diabetic nephropathy: incidence and risk factors. Diabetologia 1987;30(3):144–8.

19. Valmadrid CT, Klein R, Moss SE, et al. The risk of cardiovascular disease mortality associated with microalbuminuria and gross proteinuria in persons with older-onset diabetes mellitus. Arch Intern Med 2000; 160(8):1093–100.

20. Tonelli M, Keech A, Shepherd J, et al. Effect of pravastatin in people with diabetes and chronic kidney disease. J Am Soc Nephrol 2005;16(12): 3748–54.

21. Coresh J, Longenecker JC, Miller ER 3rd, et al. Epidemiology of cardiovascular risk factors in chronic renal disease. J Am Soc Nephrol 1998; 9(Suppl 12):S24–30.

22. Adler AI, Stevens RJ, Manley SE, et al. Development and progression of nephropathy in type 2 diabetes: the United Kingdom Prospective Diabetes Study (UKPDS 64). Kidney Int 2003;63(1):225–32.

23. Borch-Johnsen K, Andersen PK, Deckert T. The effect of proteinuria on relative mortality in type 1 (insulin-dependent) diabetes mellitus. Diabetologia 1985;28(8):590–6.

24. Dinneen SF, Gerstein HC. The association of microalbuminuria and mortality in noninsulin-dependent diabetes mellitus. A systematic overview of the literature. Arch Intern Med 1997;157(13):1413–8.

25. Fonseca VA. Risk factors for coronary heart disease in diabetes. Ann Intern Med 2000;133(2):154–6.

26. Varma R, Garrick R, McClung J, et al. Chronic renal dysfunction as an independent risk factor for the development of cardiovascular disease. Cardiol Rev 2005;13(2):98–107.

27. O'Brien T, Nguyen TT, Zimmerman BR. Hyperlipidemia and diabetes mellitus. Mayo Clin Proc 1998; 73(10):969–76.

28. Ginsberg HN. Review: efficacy and mechanisms of action of statins in the treatment of diabetic dyslipidemia. J Clin Endocrinol Metab 2006;91(2): 383–92.

29. Heart Protection Study Collaborative Group. MRC/ BHF Heart Protection Study of cholesterol lowering with simvastatin in 20,536 high-risk individuals: a randomised placebo-controlled trial. Lancet 2002; 360(9326):7–22.

30. Colhoun HM, Betteridge DJ, Durrington PN, et al. Primary prevention of cardiovascular disease with atorvastatin in type 2 diabetes in the Collaborative Atorvastatin Diabetes Study (CARDS): multicentre randomised placebo-controlled trial. Lancet 2004; 364(9435):685–96.

31. Collins R, Armitage J, Parish S, et al. MRC/BHF Heart Protection Study of cholesterol-lowering with simvastatin in 5963 people with diabetes: a randomised placebo-controlled trial. Lancet 2003; 361(9374):2005–16.

32. Cannon CP, Braunwald E, McCabe CH, et al. Intensive versus moderate lipid lowering with statins after acute coronary syndromes. N Engl J Med 2004; 350(15):1495–504.

33. LaRosa JC, Grundy SM, Waters DD, et al. Intensive lipid lowering with atorvastatin in patients with stable coronary disease. N Engl J Med 2005;352(14): 1425–35.

34. Grundy SM, Cleeman JI, Merz CN, et al. Implications of recent clinical trials for the National Cholesterol Education Program Adult Treatment Panel III Guidelines. J Am Coll Cardiol 2004;44(3):720–32.

35. Molitch ME. Management of dyslipidemias in patients with diabetes and chronic kidney disease. Clin J Am Soc Nephrol 2006;1(5):1090–9.

36. Wanner C, Krane V, Marz W, et al. Atorvastatin in patients with type 2 diabetes mellitus undergoing hemodialysis. N Engl J Med 2005;353(3):238–48.

37. Fellstrom BC, Jardine AG, Schmieder RE, et al. Rosuvastatin and cardiovascular events in patients undergoing hemodialysis. N Engl J Med 2009; 360(14):1395–407.

38. KDOQI. KDOQI Clinical Practice Guidelines and Clinical Practice Recommendations for Diabetes and Chronic Kidney Disease. Am J Kidney Dis 2007;49(2 Suppl 2):S12–154.

39. Bakris GL, Williams M, Dworkin L, et al. Preserving renal function in adults with hypertension and diabetes: a consensus approach. National Kidney Foundation Hypertension and Diabetes Executive Committees Working Group. Am J Kidney Dis Sep 2000;36(3):646–61.

40. Klag MJ, Whelton PK, Randall BL, et al. Blood pressure and end-stage renal disease in men. N Engl J Med 1996;334(1):13–8.

41. Perry HM Jr, Miller JP, Fornoff JR, et al. Early predictors of 15-year end-stage renal disease in hypertensive patients. Hypertension 1995;25(4 Pt 1):587–94.

42. Chobanian AV, Bakris GL, Black HR, et al. The Seventh Report of the Joint National Committee on Prevention, Detection, Evaluation, and Treatment of High Blood Pressure: the JNC 7 report. JAMA 2003;289(19):2560–72.

43. American Diabetes Association. Standards of medical care in diabetes–2008. Diabetes Care 2008;31(Suppl 1):S12–54.

44. Selvin E, Marinopoulos S, Berkenblit G, et al. Meta-analysis: glycosylated hemoglobin and cardiovascular disease in diabetes mellitus. Ann Intern Med 2004; 141(6):421–31.

45. Gerstein HC, Pogue J, Mann JF, et al. The relationship between dysglycaemia and cardiovascular and renal risk in diabetic and nondiabetic participants in the HOPE study: a prospective epidemiologic analysis. Diabetologia 2005;48(9):1749–55.

46. Selvin E, Coresh J, Golden SH, et al. Glycemic control and coronary heart disease risk in persons with and without diabetes: the atherosclerosis risk in communities study. Arch Intern Med 2005; 165(16):1910–6.

47. Ceriello A, Hanefeld M, Leiter L, et al. Postprandial glucose regulation and diabetic complications. Arch Intern Med 2004;164(19):2090–5.

48. DECODE Study Group, the European Diabetes Epidemiology Group. Glucose tolerance and cardiovascular mortality: comparison of fasting and 2-hour diagnostic criteria. Arch Intern Med 2001;161(3):397–405.

49. Saydah SH, Miret M, Sung J, et al. Postchallenge hyperglycemia and mortality in a national sample of U.S. adults. Diabetes Care 2001;24(8):1397–402.

50. Raz I, Wilson PW, Strojek K, et al. Effects of prandial versus fasting glycemia on cardiovascular outcomes in type 2 diabetes: the HEART2D trial. Diabetes Care 2009;32(3):381–6.

51. The effect of intensive treatment of diabetes on the development and progression of long-term complications in insulin-dependent diabetes mellitus. The Diabetes Control and Complications Trial Research Group. N Engl J Med 1993;329(14):977–86.

52. Nathan DM, Cleary PA, Backlund JY, et al. Intensive diabetes treatment and cardiovascular disease in patients with type 1 diabetes. N Engl J Med 2005; 353(25):2643–53.

53. Intensive blood-glucose control with sulphonylureas or insulin compared with conventional treatment and risk of complications in patients with type 2 diabetes (UKPDS 33). UK Prospective Diabetes Study (UKPDS) Group. Lancet 1998; 352(9131):837–53.

54. Holman RR, Paul SK, Bethel MA, et al. 10-year follow-up of intensive glucose control in type 2 diabetes. N Engl J Med 2008;359(15):1577–89.

55. Effect of intensive blood-glucose control with metformin on complications in overweight patients with type 2 diabetes (UKPDS 34). UK Prospective Diabetes Study (UKPDS) Group. Lancet 1998; 352(9131):854–65.

56. Gaede P, Vedel P, Larsen N, et al. Multifactorial intervention and cardiovascular disease in patients with type 2 diabetes. N Engl J Med 2003;348(5):383–93.

57. Gaede P, Lund-Andersen H, Parving HH, et al. Effect of a multifactorial intervention on mortality in type 2 diabetes. N Engl J Med 2008;358(6):580–91.

58. Patel A, MacMahon S, Chalmers J, et al. Intensive blood glucose control and vascular outcomes in patients with type 2 diabetes. N Engl J Med 2008; 358(24):2560–72.

59. Gerstein HC, Miller ME, Byington RP, et al. Effects of intensive glucose lowering in type 2 diabetes. N Engl J Med 2008;358(24):2545–59.

60. Duckworth W, Abraira C, Moritz T, et al. Glucose control and vascular complications in veterans with type 2 diabetes. N Engl J Med 2009;360(2):129–39.

61. Skyler JS, Bergenstal R, Bonow RO, et al. Intensive glycemic control and the prevention of cardiovascular events: implications of the ACCORD, ADVANCE, and VA Diabetes Trials: a position statement of the American Diabetes Association and a Scientific Statement of the American College of Cardiology Foundation and the American Heart Association. J Am Coll Cardiol 2009;53(3): 298–304.

62. Reaven GM. Banting lecture 1988. Role of insulin resistance in human disease. Diabetes 1988; 37(12):1595–607.

63. Frye RL, August P, Brooks MM, et al. A randomized trial of therapies for type 2 diabetes and coronary artery disease. N Engl J Med 2009; 360(24):2503–15.

The Genetics of Vascular Complications in Diabetes Mellitus

Dan Farbstein, BSc[a],*, Andrew P. Levy, MD, PhD[b]

KEYWORDS

- Diabetes • Cardiovascular disease • Polymorphism
- Genetic variance • Genotype • Phenotype

Because of increasing prevalence rates in the past decade, diabetes mellitus (DM) has become a major public health issue. Macrovascular and microvascular complications are common long-term sequelae of the disease. Cardiovascular disease (CVD) is the single most major cause of death among patients with DM, accounting for approximately 65% of mortality in DM.[1] End stage renal disease is also a major complication of DM with nearly a third of all individuals with DM eventually requiring treatment with dialysis. Overall, DM accounts for 35% of hospitalizations caused by CVD and is the leading cause of blindness in the Western world. Identification of those individuals with DM who are at greatest risk for the development of CVD would have considerable public health importance because it would allow for a more efficient allocation of resources to alleviate the burden of disease.[2] Beginning more than 20 years ago, hundreds of polymorphisms in genes that are involved in the pathogenesis of CVD and DM have been examined for their ability to predict which individuals with DM will develop CVD. These polymorphisms may modify the activity of proteins, making them more or less active, or alter their expression and stability, thus modulating their ability to retain normal vascular physiology and metabolism. **Fig. 1** provides a functional categorization of these polymorphic genes. **Table 1** provides a comprehensive list of the single-nucleotide polymorphisms (SNPs) and polymorphisms that have been assessed to date in the search for loci that may predict CVD in DM. However, only a handful of these polymorphisms have been shown reproducibly to predict diabetic CVD across various populations and ethnic groups. These polymorphisms are reviewed in this article.

PARAOXONASE

The Paraoxonase Family

Located at locus 7q21.3, the cluster of the paraoxonase (PON) gene family is comprised of three members: *PON1*, *PON2*, and *PON3*. The three members are highly homogenous, presenting with 70% similarity at the nucleotide level and 60% similarity of the amino acid sequence.[40] However, their expression patterns are varied. Although PON1 and PON3 are expressed mainly in the liver and associate with high density lipoprotein (HDL) in the circulation,[41,42] PON2 is expressed in a variety of tissues and is found on the endoplasmic reticulum and the nuclear membrane.[43] Although only PON1 exhibits the

This work was supported by grants from the United States-Israel Binational Science Foundation, Israel Science Foundation, Juvenile Diabetes Research Foundation, the Kennedy Leigh Charitable Trust, and grant RO1KD085226 from the NIH to Andrew P. Levy.
Financial Disclosure Information: Dr Levy has served in the past as a consultant for Synvista Therapeutics.
[a] Faculty of Medicine, Technion-Israel Institute of Technology, Haifa 31096, Israel
[b] Department of Cell Biology and Anatomy, Faculty of Medicine, Technion-Israel Institute of Technology, Haifa 31096, Israel
* Corresponding author.
E-mail address: dfarb@tx.technion.ac.il

Cardiol Clin 28 (2010) 477–496
doi:10.1016/j.ccl.2010.04.005
0733-8651/10/$ – see front matter © 2010 Elsevier Inc. All rights reserved.

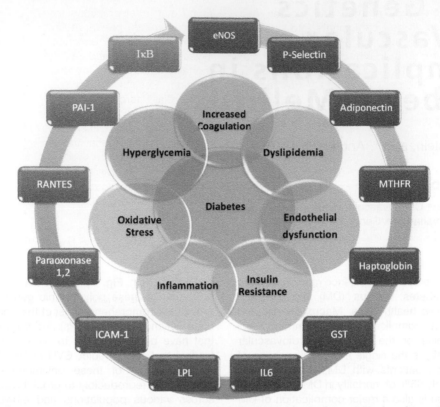

Fig. 1. Candidate genes for diabetic CVD. eNOS, endothelial nitric oxide synthase; GST, glutathione S transferase; IκB, inhibitor of NFκB; IL6, interleukin 6; LPL, lipoprotein lipase; MTHFR, methylenetetrahydrofolate reductase; PAI-1, plasminogen activator inhibitor 1; PON, paraoxonase; RANTES, regulated on activation normal T cell expressed and secreted; PAI-1, plasminogen activator inhibitor 1.

ability to hydrolyze organophosphates, the three enzymes share the ability to metabolize different lactones,[44] some of which are the product of phospholipid peroxidation.[45] It has been suggested that this enzymatic activity has a pivotal role in preserving the integrity of cell membranes, protecting it from a wide variety of endogenous and exogenous toxins. Supporting this hypothesis is the localization of PON1 to the same HDL subfraction as clusterin, which is also suspected to have a role in cell membrane protection.[46] Recently, it has been suggested that the PON enzymes have a role in innate immunity, being able to hydrolyze the quorum sensing signal molecule N-acyl-homoserine-lactone.[47]

Antiatherogenic Properties of Paraoxonase

HDL is known to attenuate the development of atherosclerosis by a variety of mechanisms, including removal of excess cholesterol from cells of the vessel wall (reverse cholesterol transport) and limiting low density lipoprotein (LDL) oxidation. These antiatherogenic activities are catalyzed by the many proteins associated with the HDL

particle. PON1 and PON3, which are associated with HDL in the plasma, take part in the antioxidant activity of HDL. PON1 diminishes LDL oxidation[48] and prevents the proinflammatory response elicited by oxidized LDL (OxLDL), the latter probably resulting from the metabolism of lipid peroxides.[49] Moreover, PON1 is critical for preventing the oxidation of HDL, allowing it to maintain its function.[50] Similar results were obtained in a study of PON1 knockout mice, where the ability of HDL isolated from these mice to limit lipid peroxidation and LDL-induced inflammation was decreased.[51] PON1 knockout mice were also more susceptible to the development of atherosclerosis in dietary or genetic models.[51,52] Demonstrating a therapeutic potential for PON1 elevation, mice overexpressing PON1 were more resistant to atherosclerosis compared with wild-type mice.[53]

Paraoxonase Genotype and Relation to Cardiovascular Disease

Genetic polymorphisms have been discovered in all the three members of the paraoxonase gene family. In PON1, which has gained the most attention concerning its relationship with CVD, several polymorphisms have been identified in coding regions, affecting the amino acid sequence, and in the promoter region. Of the polymorphisms of the promoter, the C(-107)T polymorphism has been most widely studied. Because of the differences in the affinity of the transcription factor Sp1,[54] this polymorphism has a dramatic effect on gene transcription, the -107C allele having significantly increased transcriptional activity compared with the -107T allele. This variation is reflected in higher plasma PON1 concentrations and activity in carriers of the -107C allele.[54,55] However, although significantly decreasing enzyme concentration and activity, this polymorphism has not consistently been shown to be associated with CVD.[56–59] A recent trial has shown that although the promoter polymorphisms do not affect the risk for CVD, they do influence the extent of the disease as measured by the number of coronary vessels undergoing stenosis.[58]

Of the polymorphisms in the coding region, the Glu192Arg polymorphism has gained the most interest.[60] This polymorphism results in a decrease in serum paraoxonase activity and concentration,[61] possibly caused by decreased affinity of the Arg192 polymorphism to the HDL, which leads to decreased protein stability and activity.[62] Of the many polymorphisms of the PON enzymes, the Glu192Arg polymorphism alone was found to be associated with CVD in a large meta-analysis, although the external validity of this association was questioned because of the lack of a significant association between this polymorphism and CVD in large trials and because of possible publication bias.[63] Following the many failures to associate specific polymorphisms of the PON1 gene with vascular disease, it has been suggested that the relationship between PON1 phenotype expressed by serum concentration and activity, rather than genotype, and CVD should be explored. Indeed, it has been found that PON1 activity is a predictor of CVD, regardless of PON1 genotype.[64,65] A recent large trial in which PON1 activity and genotype were tested has shown that not only do PON1 phenotype and Glu192Arg genotype determine the risk for CVD but also that the PON1 genotype is a predictor of its activity and concentration.[61]

Paraoxonase and Diabetes Mellitus

The relationship between PON1 and DM appears to be bidirectional with DM significantly decreasing PON1 concentration[66] and activity,[66–70] and in turn, PON1 genotype modulating the risk for type 2 DM.[68,71] The importance of paraoxonase activity in the prevention of DM was also demonstrated in an in vivo model, where increased PON1 expression in mice has impeded the development of streptozotocin-induced DM.[72] Similar to what is seen in non-DM individuals, PON1 concentration and activity were found to be negatively associated with CVD.[73–76] In the settings of Type 2 DM, only a single study has focused on the C-107T polymorphism, indicating an increased risk for CVD in carriers of the TT allele compared with carriers of the CT or CC alleles.[77] This genotype was also associated with decreased PON1 concentration and activity[67] and increased plasma OxLDL/apolipoprotein B (apo B) ratio among individuals with DM.[78] The Glu192Arg polymorphism was extensively studied in the settings of DM. In these settings, HDL from 192Arg allele homozygotes was less efficient in the metabolism of oxidized phospholipids,[69] although these results were contested by others showing either no difference in plasma oxidized LDL[79] or decreased oxidation in the aforementioned genotype.[80] In most epidemiologic studies, the 192Arg allele was significantly correlated with CVD,[81–84] although several studies have presented contradicting results.[74] Several studies have highlighted the importance of interaction between the PON1 Glu192Arg polymorphism and DM, arguing that this polymorphism most significantly increases the risk for CVD in the presence of DM.[85,86]

METHYLTETRAHYDROFOLATE REDUCTASE AND HOMOCYSTEINE METABOLISM
Metabolic Pathways of Homocysteine

Homocysteine (Hcy) is positioned at the crossroads of several metabolic pathways. Hcy is synthesized from methionine in a three-step reaction, which includes activation of methionine by ATP, loss of a methyl group, and enzymatic hydrolysis. Remethylation of Hcy to methionine is catalyzed by betaine-homocysteine methyltransferase in the liver or by methionine synthase (MS) in most bodily tissues, the latter depending on methyltetrahydrofolate as a methyl donor and vitamin B_{12} as a cofactor. Synthesis of methyltetrahydrofolate is catalyzed by the enzyme methylenetetrahydrofolate reductase (MTHFR) in the presence of vitamin B_2. In a state of methionine excess, Hcy is irreversibly trans-sulfurated by cystathionine β-synthase (CBS) and vitamin B_6 to cystathionine, which can be converted to cysteine.[87] A third elimination pathway of Hcy is the pathologic synthesis of the Hcy-thiolactone. This reaction is performed by methionyl-tRNA synthetase (MetRS) when Hcy is mistakenly recognized as methionine.[88]

Table 1
Single-nucleotide polymorphisms and genetic variations implicated in the risk for cardiovascular disease, in the settings of diabetes mellitus

Gene	Protein	Polymorphism	References
16p3	—		Bowden et al[3]
9p21	—	rs2383206	Doria et al[4]
ACE	Angiotensin converting enzyme	Insertion/deletion	Grammer et al[5] Burdon et al[6]
ADIPOQ/ ACDC	Adiponectin	−11391G>A	Gable et al[7]
		−11377C>G	Gable et al[7] Prior et al[8] Lacquemant et al[9]
		−11365C>G	Qi et al[10]
		−4041 A>C	Lacquemant et al[9]
		−4034A>C	Qi et al[10]
		−3964A>G	Qi et al[10]
		45T>G	Gable et al[7] Lacquemant et al[9] Qi et al[10] Vendramini et al[11] Kim et al[12] Bacci et al[13]
		276G>T	Gable et al[7] Lacquemant et al[9] Qi et al[10] Vendramini et al[11] Kim et al[12] Bacci et al[13]
		A349G	Vendramini et al[11]
		+2019 delA	Lacquemant et al[9]
ADIPOR1	Adiponectin receptor 1	rs2232853	Soccio et al[14]
		rs12733285	Soccio et al[14]
		rs1342387	Soccio et al[14]
		rs7539542	Soccio et al[14]
		rs10920531	Soccio et al[14]
		rs4950894	Soccio et al[14]
AGT	Angiotensinogen	M235T	Burdon et al[6] Lin et al[15]
AGTR1	Angiotensin-II receptor 1	T573C	Lin et al[15]
		A1166C	Lin et al[15]
AGTR1	Angiotensin receptor 1	rs5186	Burdon et al[6]
aP2	Fatty-acid binding protein	T-78C	Tuncman et al[16]
APOA4	Apolipoprotein A-IV	Gln360His	Kretowski et al[17]
		Thr347Ser	Kretowski et al[17]
APOE	Apolipoprotein E	ε2/ε3/ε4	Winkler et al[18]

Gene	Gene name	Variant	Reference
CD40	CD-40	rs1535045	Burdon et al[19]
		rs3765459	Burdon et al[19]
CD40L	CD-40 Ligand	rs3092948	Burdon et al[19]
		rs3092929	Burdon et al[19]
		rs3092923	Burdon et al[19]
		rs3092920	Burdon et al[19]
CETP	Cholesteryl ester transfer protein	rs289714	Burdon et al[20]
		I405V	Burdon et al[20]
		R451Q	Burdon et al[20]
COX2	Cyclooxygenase-2	rs689466	Rudock et al[21]
		rs20417	Rudock et al[21]
		rs2745557	Rudock et al[21]
		rs5277	Rudock et al[21]
		rs20432	Rudock et al[21]
		rs2066826	Rudock et al[21]
		rs5275	Rudock et al[21]
		rs10911902	Rudock et al[21]
CX3CR1	Fractalkine receptor	T280M	Boger et al[22]
ENPP1	Ectoenzyme nucleotide pyrophosphate phosphodiesterase 1	K121Q	Chen et al[23]
EPHX2	Epoxide hydrolase 2	rs7003694	Burdon et al[24]
		rs7837347	Burdon et al[24]
		R287Q	Burdon et al[24]
		rs721619	Burdon et al[24]
		rs747276	Burdon et al[24]
HL	Hepatic Lipase	C-480T	Burdon et al[20]
HSP70-2	Heat Shock Protein 70-2	A1267G (A/B)	Giacconi et al[25]
GCH1	GTP cyclohydrolase 1	C59038T	Liao et al[26]
GSTT1	Glutathione S transferase theta-1	1/0	Hayek et al[27]Doney et al[28]

(continued on next page)

Table 1
(continued)

Gene	Protein	Polymorphism	References
GSTM1	Glutathione S transferase mu-1	1/0	Hayek et al[27] Doney et al[28]
GSTP1	Glutathione S transferase pi-1	Ile105Val	Doney et al[28]
IL6	Interleukin 6	-174G/C	Danielsson et al[29]
LPL	Lipoprotein lipase	rs285	Burdon et al[20]
		rs320	Burdon et a l[20]
MT1A	Metallothionein 1A	A647C	Giacconi et al[30]
		A1245G	Giacconi et al[30]
MCP-1	Monocyte chemoattractant protein 1	A-2518G	Boger et al[22]
NFKBIA	Inhibitor of NFκB	A/G in the 3'-UTR	Romzova et al[31]
NFKB1	Nuclear factor κ B	CA repeat	Romzova et al[31]
NQO1	Nicotinamide adenine dinucleotide phosphate: quinone oxidoreductase 1	C609T (rs1800566)	Han et al[32]
PAI-1	Plasminogen activator inhibitor 1	−675 4G/5G insertion/ deletion	Saely et al[33]
PON2	Paraoxonase 2	S311C	Burdon et al[20]
PPARA	Peroxisome proliferator activated receptor α	L162V	Tai et al[34] Doney et al[35]
		C2528G	Doney et al[35]
P-selectin	P-selectin	Tyr715Pro	Zalewski et al[36]
		Asn562Asp	Zalewski et al[36]
		Ser290Asn	Zalewski et al[36]

Gene	Description	Variant	Reference
PTPN1	Protein tyrosine phosphatase 1B	rs2904268	Burdon et al[37]
		rs803742	Burdon et al[37]
		rs1967439	Burdon et al[37]
		rs718630	Burdon et al[37]
		rs4811078	Burdon et al[37]
		rs2206656	Burdon et al[37]
		rs932420	Burdon et al[37]
		rs3787335	Burdon et al[37]
		rs2426158	Burdon et al[37]
		rs2904269	Burdon et al[37]
		rs941798	Burdon et al[37]
		rs1570179	Burdon et al[37]
		rs3787345	Burdon et al[37]
		rs1885177	Burdon et al[37]
		rs754118	Burdon et al[37]
		rs3215684	Burdon et al[37]
		rs968701	Burdon et al[37]
		rs2282147	Burdon et al[37]
		rs718049	Burdon et al[37]
		rs718050	Burdon et al[37]
		rs3787348	Burdon et al[37]
		1484insG	Burdon et al[37]
		rs914458	Burdon et al[37]
RANTES	Regulated on activation, normal T cell expressed and secreted	A(−403)G	Boger et al[22]
		C-28G	Boger et al[22]
		In1.1C/T	Boger et al[22]
VEGF	Vascular endothelial growth factor	Insertion/Deletion	Buraczynska et al[38]
		G405C	Buraczynska et al[38]
		T(-1498)C	Suganthalakshmi et al[39]
		G(-1190)A	Suganthalakshmi et al[39]
		C(-634)G	Suganthalakshmi et al[39]
		C(-7)T	Suganthalakshmi et al[39]

Atherogenic Effects of Homocysteine

Homocysteine and its metabolites have an atherogenic potential, affecting cell survival, proliferation and apoptosis, thrombosis, and lipid metabolism and peroxidation. Hcy-thiolactone is capable of forming amide bonds with lysine residues, thus creating n-homocysteinylated proteins, altering their activity and solubility. N-homocysteinylation of the HDL-associated enzyme *PON1* that hydrolyses Hcy-thiolactone and oxidized phospholipids renders it inactive thus decreasing the antiatherogenic activity of HDL.[88] Hyperhomocysteinemia has also been associated with decreased expression of HDL-associated proteins, such as lecithin-cholesterol acyltransferase (LCAT) and apolipoprotein A-1 (apo A-1), and accelerated HDL catabolism, resulting in overall decreased HDL levels and activity.[89] Although LDL oxidation by Hcy was not proven to take place in vivo,[90] modification of apolipoprotein B-100 (apo B-100) by Hcy-thiolactone leads to its aggregation, making it cytotoxic to endothelial cells.[88] Because of the strong relationship between oxidative stress and CVD, Hcy oxidative potential has been extensively studied. A central role in Hcy-mediated oxidative stress has been attributed to its reaction with copper to produce hydrogen peroxide (H_2O_2) and other reactive oxygen species (ROS). Although Hcy promotes the synthesis of glutathione and nitrous oxide (NO), the former scavenging H_2O_2 and the latter scavenging Hcy itself, prolonged exposure to high levels of Hcy leads to saturation of these reactions, thus allowing excess Hcy to produce free H_2O_2 and ROS.[91] The pro-thrombotic effects of Hcy and its metabolites are a result of increased pro-coagulatory properties of the endothelium and decreased fibrinolysis. Treatment of endothelial cells with Hcy increased the synthesis and activation of pro-coagulatory molecules, such as tissue factor and factor V, and decreased the synthesis and activation of anticoagulatory molecules, such as heparan sulfate, protein C, NO, and prostacyclins.[91] N-homocysteinylation of fibrinogen renders it more resistant to fibrinolysis,[88] a process that is attenuated further by decreased tissue plasminogen activator activation by the endothelium.[91] Disruption of normal endothelial function by Hcy and its metabolites is not restricted to its role in coagulation and thrombolysis. Treatment with Hcy or Hcy thiolactone resulted in increased apoptosis[92] and decreased proliferation[93–95] of cultured endothelial cells. Impaired endothelial-dependent vasodilation, most likely resulting from endothelial injury, increased oxidative stress, and decreased NO bioavailability, is another manifestation of hyperhomocysteinemia.[90,91] Increased proliferation of vascular smooth muscle cells (VSMCs) occurs following exposure to Hcy.[96,97] Thickening of the vessel wall is also the result of the increased collagen production exerted by Hcy.[91]

Hyperhomocysteinemia and Cardiovascular Disease

Hyperhomocysteinemia was first implicated in the pathogenesis of vascular disease in 1969, following an observation that children carrying inherited deficiencies in the enzyme CBS presenting with homocystinuria commonly suffer from vascular diseases.[98] This observation was the cornerstone for extensive research regarding the relationship between Hcy and vascular diseases. Over the years, this relationship has been thoroughly studied with considerable evidence pointing toward a significant association between cardiovascular disease and an elevated Hcy level, which is independent of other known cardiovascular risk factors.[99–103] Consequently, Hcy-reducing treatments, generally including folate, vitamin B_6, and vitamin B_{12}, were tested for their ability to reduce the risk for CVD among individuals with hyperhomocysteinemia. Although supplementation decreases homocysteine levels, in most studies this has not been accompanied by a reduction in the risk for CVD.[102,104–106] Moreover, the results of two studies suggested a potentially harmful effect of vitamin supplementation.[107,108] An exception to these findings is the effect of folate and vitamin supplementation on stroke, where a significant risk reduction was noted.[109] It has been suggested that Hcy is only a marker of other pathologic phenomena related to CVD. However, other explanations for the discrepancy between the results of the observational studies and the clinical trials have been offered, amongst which are the duration of Hcy-lowering treatments and the confounding effect of folate fortification of grains.[110] Another possibility is that Hcy reduction may only be helpful in early stages of CVD.

Similarly to what is seen in the general population, hyperhomocysteinemia is also associated with increased CVD among patients with DM.[111–115] Although it is unclear whether hyperhomocysteinemia is one of the manifestations of DM,[116–118] in-group studies have found several correlates to Hcy levels, the most prominent being renal function.[115,118]

The Methylenetetrahydrofolate Reductase 677 CT Polymorphism

Following the discovery of the relationship between CBS deficiency, increased Hcy, and

CVD, other polymorphisms and mutations that may interfere with Hcy metabolism have been examined. The most documented polymorphism is that of the enzyme MTHFR, where a substitution of C to T occurs at position 677. This substitution results in a missense polymorphism, producing a thermolabile enzyme with decreased reactivity. The 677T allele has a frequency of 30% to 40% with 10% of all individuals homozygous for the T allele. TT homozygotes have marked hyperhomocysteinemia in states of folate deficiency.[91] Although initial studies demonstrated a strong relationship between the 677CT polymorphism and CVD,[119] these results have not been replicated[120] leading to the notion that this polymorphism may only be a minor risk factor for CVD.[121,122] The relationship between the 677 CT polymorphism and CVD in DM is also complicated. Although significant evidence exists linking the 677 CT polymorphism to diabetic retinopathy[123–125] and nephropathy,[126–128] evidence is disputed regarding its role in stroke and peripheral and coronary artery disease.[129–136]

ENDOTHELIAL NITRIC OXIDE SYNTHASE AND NITRIC OXIDE METABOLISM
Role of Nitric Oxide and Endothelial Nitric Oxide Synthase in Cardiovascular Physiology

NO has been identified as an important factor in maintaining normal cardiovascular function and preserving the integrity of the vascular bed. It inhibits thrombosis and coagulation not only by maintaining anticoagulatory and anti-thrombogenic properties of the endothelium[137] but also by inhibiting platelet activation and aggregation and thereby reducing platelet derived growth factor (PDGF)-induced proliferation of vascular smooth muscle cells in the vessel wall.[138] Acting directly on VSMCs, NO is a potent vasodilator[138] and a regulator of cell proliferation.[139] NO protects the endothelium and the underlying intima from inflammatory processes, inhibiting the expression of chemoattractants, such as monocyte chemotactic protein-1(MCP-1), and of adhesion molecules, such as vascular cell adhesion molecule 1 (VCAM-1) and intercellular adhesion molecule 1 (ICAM-1).[138] NO is also capable of acting as an antioxidant, inhibiting pro-oxidative reactions catalyzed by H_2O_2.[140]

In vivo, NO is synthesized by the nitric oxide synthase (NOS) family of enzymes. The endothelial nitric oxide synthase (eNOS) is synthesized from the gene NOS3, which is located at chromosomal locus 7q35-36.[141] Despite its name, eNOS expression is not restricted to endothelial cells and can be found in other cell types, such as erythrocytes, leukocytes, and mast cells.[137] It acts as a membrane-bound homodimer[142] catalyzing the synthesis of NO from L-arginine, a reaction that demands the presence of several cofactors, such as heme, tetrahydrobiopterin, and nicotinamide-adenine-dinucleotide phosphate.[139] The enzyme eNOS is constitutively expressed and is subjected to regulation by a variety of factors, such as calcium and calmodulin, phosphorylation, protein-protein interaction, and fatty-acid modification. Altogether, these factors determine NO production and release by the endothelium.[143]

Polymorphisms of the NOS3 Gene and Their Relation to Cardiovascular Disease

As a result of the importance of NO and eNOS in vascular physiology, polymorphisms were examined in the gene NOS3. In the coding region, the Glu298Asp (G894T) polymorphism has been most widely studied. Several studies reported differences in NO synthesis and reduced NO availability in carriers of the 298Asp variant, probably caused by protein cleavage,[144,145] but these results were contradicted by others.[146,147] Characteristics of enzymatic activity, such as K_M, V_{max}, and K_i, for various inhibitors did not differ between the 298Asp and 298Glu proteins.[147,148] In several independent studies, the 298Asp variant has been associated with poor endothelial and vasomotor function, carriers of the allele presenting with decreased flow or stimuli-dependent vasodilation,[149,150] increased coronary vascular resistance,[150] and increased vasoconstriction in response to stimuli.[151] However, these results were not observed in all trials, some finding no relation between the 298Asp allele and endothelial function.[152–154] This polymorphism has also been identified as an important determinant of collateral vessels development.[155,156]

In the promoter region, the T-786C polymorphism was identified as a predictor of eNOS expression, the -786C allele associated with decreased mRNA levels, which translates to decreased NO production[157] and decreased endothelial function.[153,158,159] The variability in mRNA expression most likely results from differential binding of an inhibitory transcription factor to the -786C allele,[158] perhaps the replication protein A1.[157]

A third polymorphism that has gained much attention is a 27 base pair tandem repeat in intron 4, where one allele, denoted a, presents with four tandem repeats and the second allele, denoted b, presents with five tandem repeats. Sparse evidence exists regarding the effect of this polymorphism on eNOS expression and activity.

Although the b allele has been linked to protein expression[160] and increased plasma NO concentrations in some[161] trials,[162–164] the allele was associated with increased specific activity.[160] Lacking a mechanism that links it with protein activity or expression, it has been suggested that this intron polymorphism is found in linkage disequilibrium with other functional polymorphisms. This theory was supported by several studies that found linkage disequilibrium between this polymorphism and the T-786C polymorphism.[160,162]

The effect of the aforementioned polymorphisms on CVD was evaluated in a recent meta-analysis. When all studies were taken into account, all three polymorphisms were found to be mild risk factors for coronary heart disease (CHD). However, when only the larger studies were examined, this association was either lost or was no longer significant.[165] In this meta-analysis, no significant association was found between these polymorphisms and other CVD outcomes, such as stroke and carotid stenosis.

NOS3 Polymorphisms and Diabetes Mellitus

Endothelial dysfunction and decreased NO bioavailability are prominent features of type 2 DM and may even appear before the onset of the disease.[166] Decreased NO release by endothelial cells may be the result of several mechanisms, including a deficiency in L-arginine, deficiencies in the various cofactors, and increased NO scavenging by ROS. Aberrant insulin signaling through the PI3K/Akt pathway in endothelial cells prevents eNOS phosphorylation on Serine 1177, thus decreasing its activity.[167] Similar to the observations in patients without DM, the evidence regarding the impact of NOS3 polymorphisms on NO production and endothelial function is inconclusive.[168–170] A limited body of data exists regarding the relationship between NOS3 polymorphisms and cardiovascular outcomes in the setting of DM. A recent review that studied the relationship between the different NOS3 polymorphisms and diabetic nephropathy was able to show a significant effect of the Glu298Asp across different populations. A specific interaction between the Glu298Asp and the 4a/b polymorphisms and severe diabetic nephropathy was shown in East Asian populations.[171] A recent meta-analysis also investigated the relationship between NOS3 polymorphism and diabetic retinopathy, failing to find a significant association between the two.[172] The relationship between the Glu298Asp polymorphism and other cardiovascular diseases in the setting of DM was identified by several,[131,173] but not all,[174,175] studies.

However, these were mostly retrospective studies with only one prospective study demonstrating such a relationship in patients with type 1 DM.[176]

HAPTOGLOBIN AND HEMOGLOBIN-MEDIATED OXIDATIVE STRESS
Haptoglobin Metabolism

Haptoglobin (Hp) is an acute-phase, plasma-born glycoprotein produced mainly by hepatocytes, most widely known for its ability to strongly bind free hemoglobin (Hb) following its release from erythrocytes.[177] The concentrations of Hp in the plasma are high, ranging from 0.3 mg/ml to 3.0 mg/ml, producing an Hp/Hb molar ratio of 400:1. This concentration allows effective scavenging of free Hb, even in the scenario of hemolysis when its levels are sharply increased.[178] In fact, Hp has a major role in iron preservation during hemolysis, as it prevents Hb filtration in the glomeruli[179] and renal damage.[180] The Hp-Hb complex is transported to the liver and other tissues to be degraded by Hp-Hb scavenger receptors, such as the CD163 receptor present on macrophages and liver Kupffer cells.[181,182] Another important aspect of Hb scavenging by Hp is the reduction in oxidative stress. Extracorpuscular Hb can initiate a free radical reaction by releasing heme iron, which acts as a potent Fenton reagent. This reaction results in the production of ROS that causes oxidative damage to their surroundings.[183] Hp binding to Hb prevents this cascade by shielding the heme iron from its aqueous surrounding.[184,185] Moreover, Hp maintains Hb integrity by preventing oxidation of the globin by heme iron, which allows effective clearance of Hb by the CD163 receptor.[186]

The Haptoglobin Polymorphism

The Hp gene has been localized to chromosome 16q22. Two Hp alleles exist in man: Hp1, with an allele frequency of 0.4; and Hp2, with an allele frequency of 0.6 in most Western populations. The alleles are found in a Hardy-Weinberg equilibrium, the frequency of the Hp1-1, Hp2-1, and Hp2-2 genotypes being 16%, 48%, and 36%, respectively.[177] The Hp2 allele, whose development most likely occurred in early human evolution, has evolved from the Hp1 allele via a duplication of exons 3 and 4 present in the Hp1 allele. Exon 3 contains a cysteine residue that can form a disulfide bridge between Hp monomers. Therefore, its duplication in the Hp2 allele makes the Hp2 protein monomer bivalent, whereas the Hp1 protein monomer is monovalent. This difference has significant implications for the stoichiometry and structure of Hp found in serum. Being monovalent, the Hp1 monomer can only bind to one other Hp molecule, forming linear dimers in the Hp1-1 genotype. The Hp2 monomer, conversely, binds two other Hp molecules and forms cyclic polymers in individuals with the Hp2-2 genotype. In the Hp2-1 genotype, heteromeric linear polymers are formed, with Hp1 proteins bracketing a chain of linear Hp2 proteins. Hp1-1 dimers may also be found in the Hp2-1 genotype.[187]

Haptoglobin Genotype and Diabetic Cardiovascular Disease: a Specific Gene-Disease Interaction

As opposed to the other CVD-related genes discussed earlier, the Hp polymorphism appears to have a unique interaction with DM. In the setting of DM, the Hp2-2 polymorphism confers a twofold to fivefold increased risk for CVD compared with the Hp1-1 and Hp2-1 genotypes.[188–192] This finding was also seen in in vivo studies where mice with Hp2-2 DM were more prone to develop retinopathy,[193] nephropathy,[194] and atherosclerosis.[195,196] In the absence of DM, the Hp1-1 genotype may be associated with increased CVD.[197,198]

Haptoglobin Polymorphism and Oxidative Stress: a Mechanism for the Gene-Disease Interaction

The underlying mechanism for the specific interaction between the Hp2-2 genotype and DM appears to be the result of its interaction with Hb. In individuals with DM, extravascular and intravascular hemolysis occur in higher rates compared with individuals without DM, thus increasing the amount of Hp-Hb molecules in plasma and tissues. As already mentioned, Hp is considered an antioxidant because of its ability to scavenge Hb and prevent the initiation of radical chain reactions. However, this antioxidant activity varies greatly between the different Hp genotypes.[184] Although the affinity for Hb is similar for Hp1-1 and Hp2-2,[199] the ability to seclude the heme-iron from its aqueous surroundings is greatly decreased in the latter. This disparity is further magnified by oxidation and glycation of Hb, both common in DM.[200] Under hyperglycemic conditions, Hp2-Hb, as compared with Hp1-Hb, evoked increased oxidative stress in cultured CD163-transfected Chinese hamster ovary cells.[200] In vivo, the ability of Hp1-1 to better shield Hb is translated to a decrease in redox active heme iron in Hp1-1 DM compared with mice and humans with Hp2-2 DM, both in blood and tissues.[200,201] The increase in plasma oxidative stress in individuals with Hp2-2 is also indicated

by the decrease in antioxidants, such as vitamin C,[187] in the serum of individuals with Hp2-2. Furthermore, increased oxidative stress and hyperglycemia lead to decreased expression of CD163 on macrophages by inducing its shedding and decreasing transcription.[202,203] Finally, clearance rate of the Hp-Hb-2-2 complex by the CD163 receptor is decreased compared with Hp-Hb-1-1, prolonging its presence in tissues[199] and perhaps decreasing the expression of CD163 itself.[204]

Another novel aspect of Hp-Hb-2-2 mediated oxidative stress is related to the association of Hp with HDL. Hp, either free or Hb-bound, is a member of the HDL proteome.[205] Because the Hp2-2 polymers contain more Hp monomers than the Hp1-1 dimers, Hp is more abundant in the HDL of individuals with Hp2-2.[205] In individuals with Hp2-2 DM, as a result of the impaired clearance of Hp-Hb, there is an increased binding of Hp-Hb to HDL, which along with the decreased antioxidant properties of Hp 2-2, expose HDL particles of individuals with Hp2-2 DM to increased oxidative stress, expressed by an increase in HDL-associated lipid peroxides. This oxidative modification of HDL in individuals with Hp2-2 DM results in a decrease in HDL-related functions, such as reverse cholesterol efflux and cholesterol esterification,[195,205] and paradoxically may result in the transformation of the HDL particle in individuals with Hp2-2 DM into a proatherogenic species. This pathway may form the basis for the pharmacogenetic relationship between vitamin E and the Hp2-2 genotype whereby vitamin E can markedly reduce CVD in individuals with Hp2-2 DM, which was recently reviewed.[206,207]

SUMMARY AND FUTURE PERSPECTIVES

With the advent of genome-wide association studies, hundreds of genetic polymorphisms with a possible impact on diabetic CVD are being investigated. However, most of these polymorphisms have failed to show any significant effect when tested across various populations. These findings are caused by the nature of the polymorphisms being tested, which are usually SNPs that have no established effect on protein activity or expression. Such polymorphisms are likely in linkage disequilibrium with other genetic markers that directly alter disease progression and therefore these SNP-disease associations may not be preserved in all populations and may be subject to population stratification. Polymorphisms in the Hp or PON genes discussed here do not suffer from this setback. Having a direct effect on the pathophysiology of the disease, the Hp and PON polymorphisms are risk factors for CVD in diverse populations.

Genetic testing certainly portends to be an important component of personalized medicine, but only when it can be accompanied by a treatment plan that would match the genetic profile of patients. Although such treatment plans may include more aggressive treatment to at-risk individuals, they may also include more frequent screening and closer monitoring, as is customarily done for carriers of genetic mutations associated with increased risk for cancer. In addition, as illustrated by the pharmacogenomic interaction between the Hp genotype and vitamin E on CVD risk,[206,207] these genetic markers might be useful in the identification of which individuals may benefit from specific drug treatments.

REFERENCES

1. American Diabetes Association. Economic costs of diabetes in the U.S. in 2007. Diabetes Care 2008; 31(3):596–615.

2. Levy AP. Application of pharmacogenomics in the prevention of diabetic cardiovascular disease: mechanistic basis and clinical evidence for utilization of the haptoglobin genotype in determining benefit from antioxidant therapy. Pharmacol Ther 2006;112(2):501–12.

3. Bowden DW, Lehtinen AB, Ziegler JT, et al. Genetic epidemiology of subclinical cardiovascular disease in the diabetes heart study. Ann Hum Genet 2008; 72(Pt 5):598–610.

4. Doria A, Wojcik J, Xu R, et al. Interaction between poor glycemic control and 9p21 locus on risk of coronary artery disease in type 2 diabetes. JAMA 2008;300(20):2389–97.

5. Grammer TB, Renner W, von Karger S, et al. The angiotensin-I converting enzyme I/D polymorphism is not associated with type 2 diabetes in individuals undergoing coronary angiography. (The Ludwigshafen Risk and Cardiovascular Health Study). Mol Genet Metab 2006;88(4):378–83.

6. Burdon KP, Langefeld CD, Wagenknecht LE, et al. Association analysis of genes in the renin-angiotensin system with subclinical cardiovascular disease in families with Type 2 diabetes mellitus: the Diabetes Heart Study. Diabet Med 2006;23(3): 228–34.

7. Gable DR, Matin J, Whittall R, et al. Common adiponectin gene variants show different effects on risk of cardiovascular disease and type 2 diabetes in European subjects. Ann Hum Genet 2007;71(Pt 4): 453–66.

8. Prior SL, Gable DR, Cooper JA, et al. Association between the adiponectin promoter rs266729 gene variant and oxidative stress in patients with diabetes mellitus. Eur Heart J 2009;30(10):1263–9.

9. Lacquemant C, Froguel P, Lobbens S, et al. The adiponectin gene SNP+45 is associated with coronary artery disease in Type 2 (non-insulin-dependent) diabetes mellitus. Diabet Med 2004;21(7):776–81.

10. Qi L, Doria A, Manson JE, et al. Adiponectin genetic variability, plasma adiponectin, and cardiovascular risk in patients with type 2 diabetes. Diabetes 2006;55(5):1512–6.

11. Vendramini MF, Pereira AC, Ferreira SR, et al. Association of genetic variants in the adiponectin encoding gene (ADIPOQ) with type 2 diabetes in Japanese Brazilians. J Diabetes Complications 2010;24(2):115–20.

12. Kim SH, Kang ES, Hur KY, et al. Adiponectin gene polymorphism 45T>G is associated with carotid artery plaques in patients with type 2 diabetes mellitus. Metabolism 2008;57(2):274–9.

13. Bacci S, Menzaghi C, Ercolino T, et al. The +276 G/T single nucleotide polymorphism of the adiponectin gene is associated with coronary artery disease in type 2 diabetic patients. Diabetes Care 2004; 27(8):2015–20.

14. Soccio T, Zhang YY, Bacci S, et al. Common haplotypes at the adiponectin receptor 1 (ADIPOR1) locus are associated with increased risk of coronary artery disease in type 2 diabetes. Diabetes 2006;55(10):2763–70.

15. Lin J, Hu FB, Qi L, et al. Genetic polymorphisms of angiotensin-2 type 1 receptor and angiotensinogen and risk of renal dysfunction and coronary heart disease in type 2 diabetes mellitus. BMC Nephrol 2009;10:9.

16. Tuncman G, Erbay E, Hom X, et al. A genetic variant at the fatty acid-binding protein aP2 locus reduces the risk for hypertriglyceridemia, type 2 diabetes, and cardiovascular disease. Proc Natl Acad Sci U S A 2006;103(18):6970–5.

17. Kretowski A, Hokanson JE, McFann K, et al. The apolipoprotein A-IV Gln360His polymorphism predicts progression of coronary artery calcification in patients with type 1 diabetes. Diabetologia 2006;49(8):1946–54.

18. Winkler K, Hoffmann MM, Krane V, et al. Apolipoprotein E genotype predicts cardiovascular endpoints in dialysis patients with type 2 diabetes mellitus. Atherosclerosis 2009;208(1):197–202.

19. Burdon KP, Langefeld CD, Beck SR, et al. Variants of the CD40 gene but not of the CD40L gene are associated with coronary artery calcification in the Diabetes Heart Study (DHS). Am Heart J 2006; 151(3):706–11.

20. Burdon KP, Langefeld CD, Beck SR, et al. Association of genes of lipid metabolism with measures of subclinical cardiovascular disease in the Diabetes Heart Study. J Med Genet 2005;42(9):720–4.

21. Rudock ME, Liu Y, Ziegler JT, et al. Association of polymorphisms in cyclooxygenase (COX)-2 with coronary and carotid calcium in the Diabetes Heart Study. Atherosclerosis 2009;203(2):459–65.

22. Boger CA, Fischereder M, Deinzer M, et al. RANTES gene polymorphisms predict all-cause and cardiac mortality in type 2 diabetes mellitus hemodialysis patients. Atherosclerosis 2005; 183(1):121–9.

23. Chen MP, Chung FM, Chang DM, et al. ENPP1 K121Q polymorphism is not related to type 2 diabetes mellitus, features of metabolic syndrome, and diabetic cardiovascular complications in a Chinese population. Rev Diabet Stud 2006; 3(1):21–30.

24. Burdon KP, Lehtinen AB, Langefeld CD, et al. Genetic analysis of the soluble epoxide hydrolase gene, EPHX2, in subclinical cardiovascular disease in the Diabetes Heart Study. Diab Vasc Dis Res 2008;5(2):128–34.

25. Giacconi R, Caruso C, Lio D, et al. 1267 HSP70-2 polymorphism as a risk factor for carotid plaque rupture and cerebral ischaemia in old type 2 diabetes-atherosclerotic patients. Mech Ageing Dev 2005;126(8):866–73.

26. Liao YF, Zeng TS, Chen LL, et al. Association of a functional polymorphism (C59038T) in GTP cyclohydrolase 1 gene and Type 2 diabetic macrovascular disease in the Chinese population. J Diabetes Complications Jun 8 2009 [Online].

27. Hayek T, Stephens JW, Hubbart CS, et al. A common variant in the glutathione S transferase gene is associated with elevated markers of inflammation and lipid peroxidation in subjects with diabetes mellitus. Atherosclerosis 2006; 184(2):404–12.

28. Doney AS, Lee S, Leese GP, et al. Increased cardiovascular morbidity and mortality in type 2 diabetes is associated with the glutathione S transferase theta-null genotype: a Go-DARTS study. Circulation 2005;111(22):2927–34.

29. Danielsson P, Truedsson L, Eriksson KF, et al. Inflammatory markers and IL-6 polymorphism in peripheral arterial disease with and without diabetes mellitus. Vasc Med 2005;10(3):191–8.

30. Giacconi R, Bonfigli AR, Testa R, et al. +647 A/C and +1245 MT1A polymorphisms in the susceptibility of diabetes mellitus and cardiovascular complications. Mol Genet Metab 2008;94(1): 98–104.

31. Romzova M, Hohenadel D, Kolostova K, et al. NFkappaB and its inhibitor IkappaB in relation to type 2 diabetes and its microvascular and atherosclerotic complications. Hum Immunol 2006;67(9): 706–13.

32. Han SJ, Kang ES, Kim HJ, et al. The C609T variant of NQO1 is associated with carotid artery plaques in patients with type 2 diabetes. Mol Genet Metab 2009;97(1):85–90.

33. Saely CH, Muendlein A, Vonbank A, et al. Type 2 diabetes significantly modulates the cardiovascular risk conferred by the PAI-1 -675 4G/5G polymorphism in angiographied coronary patients. Clin Chim Acta 2008;396(1–2):18–22.

34. Tai ES, Collins D, Robins SJ, et al. The L162V polymorphism at the peroxisome proliferator activated receptor alpha locus modulates the risk of cardiovascular events associated with insulin resistance and diabetes mellitus: the Veterans Affairs HDL Intervention Trial (VA-HIT). Atherosclerosis 2006; 187(1):153–60.

35. Doney AS, Fischer B, Lee SP, et al. Association of common variation in the PPARA gene with incident myocardial infarction in individuals with type 2 diabetes: a Go-DARTS study. Nucl Recept 2005;3:4.

36. Zalewski G, Ciccarone E, Di Castelnuovo A, et al. P-selectin gene genotypes or haplotypes and cardiovascular complications in type 2 diabetes mellitus. Nutr Metab Cardiovasc Dis 2006;16(6): 418–25.

37. Burdon KP, Bento JL, Langefeld CD, et al. Association of protein tyrosine phosphatase-N1 polymorphisms with coronary calcified plaque in the Diabetes Heart Study. Diabetes 2006;55(3):651–8.

38. Buraczynska M, Ksiazek P, Baranowicz-Gaszczyk I, et al. Association of the VEGF gene polymorphism with diabetic retinopathy in type 2 diabetes patients. Nephrol Dial Transplant 2007; 22(3):827–32.

39. Suganthalakshmi B, Anand R, Kim R, et al. Association of VEGF and eNOS gene polymorphisms in type 2 diabetic retinopathy. Mol Vis 2006;12: 336–41.

40. Primo-Parmo SL, Sorenson RC, Teiber J, et al. The human serum paraoxonase/arylesterase gene (PON1) is one member of a multigene family. Genomics 1996;33(3):498–507.

41. Blatter MC, James RW, Messmer S, et al. Identification of a distinct human high-density lipoprotein subspecies defined by a lipoprotein-associated protein, K-45. Identity of K-45 with paraoxonase. Eur J Biochem 1993;211(3):871–9.

42. Reddy ST, Wadleigh DJ, Grijalva V, et al. Human paraoxonase-3 is an HDL-associated enzyme with biological activity similar to paraoxonase-1 protein but is not regulated by oxidized lipids. Arterioscler Thromb Vasc Biol 2001;21(4):542–7.

43. Ng CJ, Wadleigh DJ, Gangopadhyay A, et al. Paraoxonase-2 is a ubiquitously expressed protein with antioxidant properties and is capable of preventing cell-mediated oxidative modification of low density lipoprotein. J Biol Chem 2001;276(48):44444–9.

44. Draganov DI, Teiber JF, Speelman A, et al. Human paraoxonases (PON1, PON2, and PON3) are

lactonases with overlapping and distinct substrate specificities. J Lipid Res 2005;46(6):1239–47.

45. Shih DM, Lusis AJ. The roles of PON1 and PON2 in cardiovascular disease and innate immunity. Curr Opin Lipidol 2009;20(4):288–92.

46. Durrington PN, Mackness B, Mackness MI. Paraoxonase and atherosclerosis. Arterioscler Thromb Vasc Biol 2001;21(4):473–80.

47. Yang F, Wang LH, Wang J, et al. Quorum quenching enzyme activity is widely conserved in the sera of mammalian species. FEBS Lett 2005;579(17): 3713–7.

48. Mackness MI, Arrol S, Durrington PN. Paraoxonase prevents accumulation of lipoperoxides in low-density lipoprotein. FEBS Lett 1991;286(1–2): 152–4.

49. Watson AD, Berliner JA, Hama SY, et al. Protective effect of high density lipoprotein associated paraoxonase. Inhibition of the biological activity of minimally oxidized low density lipoprotein. J Clin Invest 1995;96(6):2882–91.

50. Aviram M, Rosenblat M, Bisgaier CL, et al. Paraoxonase inhibits high-density lipoprotein oxidation and preserves its functions. A possible peroxidative role for paraoxonase. J Clin Invest 1998; 101(8):1581–90.

51. Shih DM, Gu L, Xia YR, et al. Mice lacking serum paraoxonase are susceptible to organophosphate toxicity and atherosclerosis. Nature 1998; 394(6690):284–7.

52. Shih DM, Xia YR, Wang XP, et al. Combined serum paraoxonase knockout/apolipoprotein E knockout mice exhibit increased lipoprotein oxidation and atherosclerosis. J Biol Chem 2000;275(23):17527–35.

53. Tward A, Xia YR, Wang XP, et al. Decreased atherosclerotic lesion formation in human serum paraoxonase transgenic mice. Circulation 2002;106(4): 484–90.

54. Deakin S, Leviev I, Brulhart-Meynet MC, et al. Paraoxonase-1 promoter haplotypes and serum paraoxonase: a predominant role for polymorphic position - 107, implicating the Sp1 transcription factor. Biochem J 2003;372(Pt 2):643–9.

55. Leviev I, James RW. Promoter polymorphisms of human paraoxonase PON1 gene and serum paraoxonase activities and concentrations. Arterioscler Thromb Vasc Biol 2000;20(2):516–21.

56. Leviev I, Righetti A, James RW. Paraoxonase promoter polymorphism T(-107)C and relative paraoxonase deficiency as determinants of risk of coronary artery disease. J Mol Med 2001;79(8): 457–63.

57. Wang X, Fan Z, Huang J, et al. Extensive association analysis between polymorphisms of PON gene cluster with coronary heart disease in Chinese Han population. Arterioscler Thromb Vasc Biol 2003; 23(2):328–34.

58. Najafi M, Gohari LH, Firoozrai M. Paraoxonase 1 gene promoter polymorphisms are associated with the extent of stenosis in coronary arteries. Thromb Res 2009;123(3):503–10.

59. Yamada Y, Izawa H, Ichihara S, et al. Prediction of the risk of myocardial infarction from polymorphisms in candidate genes. N Engl J Med 2002; 347(24):1916–23.

60. Adkins S, Gan KN, Mody M, et al. Molecular basis for the polymorphic forms of human serum paraoxonase/arylesterase: glutamine or arginine at position 191, for the respective A or B allozymes. Am J Hum Genet 1993;52(3):598–608.

61. Bhattacharyya T, Nicholls SJ, Topol EJ, et al. Relationship of paraoxonase 1 (PON1) gene polymorphisms and functional activity with systemic oxidative stress and cardiovascular risk. JAMA 2008;299(11):1265–76.

62. Gaidukov L, Rosenblat M, Aviram M, et al. The 192R/Q polymorphs of serum paraoxonase PON1 differ in HDL binding, lipolactonase stimulation, and cholesterol efflux. J Lipid Res 2006;47(11): 2492–502.

63. Wheeler JG, Keavney BD, Watkins H, et al. Four paraoxonase gene polymorphisms in 11212 cases of coronary heart disease and 12786 controls: meta-analysis of 43 studies. Lancet 2004; 363(9410):689–95.

64. Jarvik GP, Hatsukami TS, Carlson C, et al. Paraoxonase activity, but not haplotype utilizing the linkage disequilibrium structure, predicts vascular disease. Arterioscler Thromb Vasc Biol 2003; 23(8):1465–71.

65. Mackness B, Davies GK, Turkie W, et al. Paraoxonase status in coronary heart disease: are activity and concentration more important than genotype? Arterioscler Thromb Vasc Biol 2001;21(9):1451–7.

66. Mackness B, Mackness MI, Arrol S, et al. Serum paraoxonase (PON1) 55 and 192 polymorphism and paraoxonase activity and concentration in non-insulin dependent diabetes mellitus. Atherosclerosis 1998;139(2):341–9.

67. Inoue M, Suehiro T, Nakamura T, et al. Serum arylesterase/diazoxonase activity and genetic polymorphisms in patients with type 2 diabetes. Metabolism 2000;49(11):1400–5.

68. Flekac M, Skrha J, Zidkova K, et al. Paraoxonase 1 gene polymorphisms and enzyme activities in diabetes mellitus. Physiol Res 2008;57(5):717–26.

69. Mastorikou M, Mackness M, Mackness B. Defective metabolism of oxidized phospholipid by HDL from people with type 2 diabetes. Diabetes 2006; 55(11):3099–103.

70. Mackness B, Durrington PN, Boulton AJ, et al. Serum paraoxonase activity in patients with type 1 diabetes compared to healthy controls. Eur J Clin Invest 2002;32(4):259–64.

71. van den Berg SW, Jansen EH, Kruijshoop M, et al. Paraoxonase 1 phenotype distribution and activity differs in subjects with newly diagnosed Type 2 diabetes (the CODAM Study). Diabet Med 2008; 25(2):186–93.

72. Rozenberg O, Shiner M, Aviram M, et al. Paraoxonase 1 (PON1) attenuates diabetes development in mice through its antioxidative properties. Free Radic Biol Med 2008;44(11):1951–9.

73. Ikeda Y, Inoue M, Suehiro T, et al. Low human paraoxonase predicts cardiovascular events in Japanese patients with type 2 diabetes. Acta Diabetol 2009;46(3):239–42.

74. Mackness B, Durrington PN, Abuashia B, et al. Low paraoxonase activity in type II diabetes mellitus complicated by retinopathy. Clin Sci (Lond) 2000; 98(3):355–63.

75. Kosaka T, Yamaguchi M, Motomura T, et al. Investigation of the relationship between atherosclerosis and paraoxonase or homocysteine thiolactonase activity in patients with type 2 diabetes mellitus using a commercially available assay. Clin Chim Acta 2005;359(1–2):156–62.

76. Ikeda Y, Suehiro T, Inoue M, et al. Serum paraoxonase activity and its relationship to diabetic complications in patients with non-insulin-dependent diabetes mellitus. Metabolism 1998;47(5): 598–602.

77. James RW, Leviev I, Ruiz J, et al. Promoter polymorphism T(-107)C of the paraoxonase PON1 gene is a risk factor for coronary heart disease in type 2 diabetic patients. Diabetes 2000;49(8):1390–3.

78. Tsuzura S, Ikeda Y, Suehiro T, et al. Correlation of plasma oxidized low-density lipoprotein levels to vascular complications and human serum paraoxonase in patients with type 2 diabetes. Metabolism 2004;53(3):297–302.

79. Sampson MJ, Braschi S, Willis G, et al. Paraoxonase-1 (PON-1) genotype and activity and in vivo oxidized plasma low-density lipoprotein in type II diabetes. Clin Sci (Lond) 2005;109(2):189–97.

80. Agachan B, Yilmaz H, Ergen HA, et al. Paraoxonase (PON1) 55 and 192 polymorphism and its effects to oxidant-antioxidant system in Turkish patients with type 2 diabetes mellitus. Physiol Res 2005;54(3):287–93.

81. Pfohl M, Koch M, Enderle MD, et al. Paraoxonase 192 Gln/Arg gene polymorphism, coronary artery disease, and myocardial infarction in type 2 diabetes. Diabetes 1999;48(3):623–7.

82. Murata M, Maruyama T, Suzuki Y, et al. Paraoxonase 1 Gln/Arg polymorphism is associated with the risk of microangiopathy in type 2 diabetes mellitus. Diabet Med 2004;21(8):837–44.

83. Odawara M, Tachi Y, Yamashita K. Paraoxonase polymorphism (Gln192-Arg) is associated with coronary heart disease in Japanese noninsulin-dependent diabetes mellitus. J Clin Endocrinol Metab 1997;82(7):2257–60.

84. Ruiz J, Blanche H, James RW, et al. Gln-Arg192 polymorphism of paraoxonase and coronary heart disease in type 2 diabetes. Lancet 1995; 346(8979):869–72.

85. Aubo C, Senti M, Marrugat J, et al. Risk of myocardial infarction associated with Gln/Arg 192 polymorphism in the human paraoxonase gene and diabetes mellitus. The REGICOR Investigators. Eur Heart J 2000;21(1):33–8.

86. Li J, Wang X, Huo Y, et al. PON1 polymorphism, diabetes mellitus, obesity, and risk of myocardial infarction: modifying effect of diabetes mellitus and obesity on the association between PON1 polymorphism and myocardial infarction. Genet Med 2005;7(1):58–63.

87. Finkelstein JD. Methionine metabolism in mammals. J Nutr Biochem 1990;1(5):228–37.

88. Jakubowski H. The pathophysiological hypothesis of homocysteine thiolactone-mediated vascular disease. J Physiol Pharmacol 2008;59(Suppl 9): 155–67.

89. Obeid R, Herrmann W. Homocysteine and lipids: S-adenosyl methionine as a key intermediate. FEBS Lett 2009;583(8):1215–25.

90. Refsum H, Ueland PM, Nygard O, et al. Homocysteine and cardiovascular disease. Annu Rev Med 1998;49:31–62.

91. Nygard O, Vollset SE, Refsum H, et al. Total homocysteine and cardiovascular disease. J Intern Med 1999;246(5):425–54.

92. Kerkeni M, Tnani M, Chuniaud L, et al. Comparative study on in vitro effects of homocysteine thiolactone and homocysteine on HUVEC cells: evidence for a stronger proapoptotic and proinflammative homocysteine thiolactone. Mol Cell Biochem 2006;291(1–2):119–26.

93. Chang PY, Lu SC, Lee CM, et al. Homocysteine inhibits arterial endothelial cell growth through transcriptional downregulation of fibroblast growth factor-2 involving G protein and DNA methylation. Circ Res 2008;102(8):933–41.

94. Jamaluddin MD, Chen I, Yang F, et al. Homocysteine inhibits endothelial cell growth via DNA hypomethylation of the cyclin A gene. Blood 2007; 110(10):3648–55.

95. Wang H, Yoshizumi M, Lai K, et al. Inhibition of growth and p21ras methylation in vascular endothelial cells by homocysteine but not cysteine. J Biol Chem 1997;272(40):25380–5.

96. Tsai JC, Wang H, Perrella MA, et al. Induction of cyclin A gene expression by homocysteine in vascular smooth muscle cells. J Clin Invest 1996; 97(1):146–53.

97. Tsai JC, Perrella MA, Yoshizumi M, et al. Promotion of vascular smooth muscle cell growth by

homocysteine: a link to atherosclerosis. Proc Natl Acad Sci U S A 1994;91(14):6369–73.

98. McCully KS. Vascular pathology of homocysteinemia: implications for the pathogenesis of arteriosclerosis. Am J Pathol 1969;56(1):111–28.

99. Khandanpour N, Loke YK, Meyer FJ, et al. Homocysteine and peripheral arterial disease: systematic review and meta-analysis. Eur J Vasc Endovasc Surg 2009;38(3):316–22.

100. Humphrey LL, Fu R, Rogers K, et al. Homocysteine level and coronary heart disease incidence: a systematic review and meta-analysis. Mayo Clin Proc 2008;83(11):1203–12.

101. Homocysteine Studies Collaboration. Homocysteine and risk of ischemic heart disease and stroke: a meta-analysis. JAMA 2002;288(16):2015–22.

102. Mager A, Orvin K, Koren-Morag N, et al. Impact of homocysteine-lowering vitamin therapy on long-term outcome of patients with coronary artery disease. Am J Cardiol 2009;104(6):745–9.

103. Van Guelpen B, Hultdin J, Johansson I, et al. Plasma folate and total homocysteine levels are associated with the risk of myocardial infarction, independently of each other and of renal function. J Intern Med 2009;266(2):182–95.

104. Albert CM, Cook NR, Gaziano JM, et al. Effect of folic acid and B vitamins on risk of cardiovascular events and total mortality among women at high risk for cardiovascular disease: a randomized trial. JAMA 2008;299(17):2027–36.

105. Bazzano LA, Reynolds K, Holder KN, et al. Effect of folic acid supplementation on risk of cardiovascular diseases: a meta-analysis of randomized controlled trials. JAMA 2006;296(22):2720–6.

106. Ebbing M, Bleie O, Ueland PM, et al. Mortality and cardiovascular events in patients treated with homocysteine-lowering B vitamins after coronary angiography: a randomized controlled trial. JAMA 2008;300(7):795–804.

107. Bonaa KH, Njolstad I, Ueland PM, et al. Homocysteine lowering and cardiovascular events after acute myocardial infarction. N Engl J Med 2006; 354(15):1578–88.

108. Lonn E, Yusuf S, Arnold MJ, et al. Homocysteine lowering with folic acid and B vitamins in vascular disease. N Engl J Med 2006;354(15):1567–77.

109. Wang X, Qin X, Demirtas H, et al. Efficacy of folic acid supplementation in stroke prevention: a meta-analysis. Lancet 2007;369(9576):1876–82.

110. Carlsson CM. Lowering homocysteine for stroke prevention. Lancet 2007;369(9576):1841–2.

111. Kark JD, Selhub J, Bostom A, et al. Plasma homocysteine and all-cause mortality in diabetes. Lancet 1999;353(9168):1936–7.

112. Hoogeveen EK, Kostense PJ, Beks PJ, et al. Hyperhomocysteinemia is associated with an increased risk of cardiovascular disease, especially in non-insulin-dependent diabetes mellitus: a population-based study. Arterioscler Thromb Vasc Biol 1998;18(1):133–8.

113. Brazionis L, Rowley K Sr, Itsiopoulos C, et al. Homocysteine and diabetic retinopathy. Diabetes Care 2008;31(1):50–6.

114. Becker A, Kostense PJ, Bos G, et al. Hyperhomocysteinaemia is associated with coronary events in type 2 diabetes. J Intern Med 2003;253(3): 293–300.

115. Buysschaert M, Dramais AS, Wallemacq PE, et al. Hyperhomocysteinemia in type 2 diabetes: relationship to macroangiopathy, nephropathy, and insulin resistance. Diabetes Care 2000;23(12): 1816–22.

116. Mazza A, Bossone E, Mazza F, et al. Reduced serum homocysteine levels in type 2 diabetes. Nutr Metab Cardiovasc Dis 2005;15(2):118–24.

117. Ndrepepa G, Kastrati A, Braun S, et al. Circulating homocysteine levels in patients with type 2 diabetes mellitus. Nutr Metab Cardiovasc Dis 2008; 18(1):66–73.

118. Emoto M, Kanda H, Shoji T, et al. Impact of insulin resistance and nephropathy on homocysteine in type 2 diabetes. Diabetes Care 2001;24(3):533–8.

119. Kluijtmans LA, van den Heuvel LP, Boers GH, et al. Molecular genetic analysis in mild hyperhomocysteinemia: a common mutation in the methylenetetrahydrofolate reductase gene is a genetic risk factor for cardiovascular disease. Am J Hum Genet 1996;58(1):35–41.

120. Deloughery TG, Evans A, Sadeghi A, et al. Common mutation in methylenetetrahydrofolate reductase. Correlation with homocysteine metabolism and late-onset vascular disease. Circulation 1996;94(12):3074–8.

121. Lewis SJ, Ebrahim S, Davey Smith G. Meta-analysis of MTHFR 677C->T polymorphism and coronary heart disease: does totality of evidence support causal role for homocysteine and preventive potential of folate? BMJ 2005; 331(7524):1053.

122. Khandanpour N, Willis G, Meyer FJ, et al. Peripheral arterial disease and methylenetetrahydrofolate reductase (MTHFR) C677T mutations: a case-control study and meta-analysis. J Vasc Surg 2009;49(3):711–8.

123. Sun J, Xu Y, Zhu Y, et al. The relationship between MTHFR gene polymorphisms, plasma homocysteine levels and diabetic retinopathy in type 2 diabetes mellitus. Chin Med J (Engl) 2003;116(1):145–7.

124. Maeda M, Yamamoto I, Fukuda M, et al. MTHFR gene polymorphism is susceptible to diabetic retinopathy but not to diabetic nephropathy in Japanese type 2 diabetic patients. J Diabetes Complications 2008;22(2):119–25.

125. Maeda M, Yamamoto I, Fukuda M, et al. MTHFR gene polymorphism as a risk factor for diabetic retinopathy in type 2 diabetic patients without serum creatinine elevation. Diabetes Care 2003; 26(2):547–8.

126. Moczulski D, Fojcik H, Zukowska-Szczechowska E, et al. Effects of the C677T and A1298C polymorphisms of the MTHFR gene on the genetic predisposition for diabetic nephropathy. Nephrol Dial Transplant 2003;18(8):1535–40.

127. Ukinc K, Ersoz HO, Karahan C, et al. Methyltetrahydrofolate reductase C677T gene mutation and hyperhomocysteinemia as a novel risk factor for diabetic nephropathy. Endocrine 2009;36(2):255–61.

128. Sun J, Xu Y, Zhu Y, et al. Genetic polymorphism of methylenetetrahydrofolate reductase as a risk factor for diabetic nephropathy in Chinese type 2 diabetic patients. Diabetes Res Clin Pract 2004; 64(3):185–90.

129. Mazza A, Motti C, Nulli A, et al. Lack of association between carotid intima-media thickness and methylenetetrahydrofolate reductase gene polymorphism or serum homocysteine in non-insulin-dependent diabetes mellitus. Metabolism 2000; 49(6):718–23.

130. Hermans MP, Gala JL, Buysschaert M. The MTHFR CT polymorphism confers a high risk for stroke in both homozygous and heterozygous T allele carriers with Type 2 diabetes. Diabet Med 2006; 23(5):529–36.

131. Szabo GV, Kunstar A, Acsady G. Methylentetrahydrofolate Reductase and Nitric Oxide Synthase Polymorphism in Patients with Atherosclerosis and Diabetes. Pathol Oncol Res 2009;15(4):631–7.

132. Mazza A, Motti C, Nulli A, et al. Serum homocysteine, MTHFR gene polymorphism, and carotid intimal-medial thickness in NIDDM subjects. J Thromb Thrombolysis 1999;8(3):207–12.

133. Kaye JM, Stanton KG, McCann VJ, et al. Homocysteine, folate, methylene tetrahydrofolate reductase genotype and vascular morbidity in diabetic subjects. Clin Sci (Lond) 2002;102(6): 631–7.

134. Pollex RL, Mamakeesick M, Zinman B, et al. Methylenetetrahydrofolate reductase polymorphism 677C>T is associated with peripheral arterial disease in type 2 diabetes. Cardiovasc Diabetol 2005;4:17.

135. Sun J, Xu Y, Xue J, et al. Methylenetetrahydrofolate reductase polymorphism associated with susceptibility to coronary heart disease in Chinese type 2 diabetic patients. Mol Cell Endocrinol 2005; 229(1–2):95–101.

136. Russo GT, Di Benedetto A, Magazzu D, et al. Mild hyperhomocysteinemia, C677T polymorphism on methylenetetrahydrofolate reductase gene and the risk of macroangiopathy in type 2 diabetes: a prospective study. Acta Diabetol 2009 [Online].

137. Dudzinski DM, Michel T. Life history of eNOS: partners and pathways. Cardiovasc Res 2007;75(2): 247–60.

138. Li H, Forstermann U. Nitric oxide in the pathogenesis of vascular disease. J Pathol 2000;190(3): 244–54.

139. Napoli C, Ignarro LJ. Nitric oxide and pathogenic mechanisms involved in the development of vascular diseases. Arch Pharm Res 2009;32(8): 1103–8.

140. Kagan VE, Laskin JD. Direct and indirect antioxidant effects of nitric oxide: radically unsettled issues. Antioxid Redox Signal 2001;3(2):173–5.

141. Marsden PA, Heng HH, Scherer SW, et al. Structure and chromosomal localization of the human constitutive endothelial nitric oxide synthase gene. J Biol Chem 1993;268(23):17478–88.

142. Andrew PJ, Mayer B. Enzymatic function of nitric oxide synthases. Cardiovasc Res 1999;43(3):521–31.

143. Napoli C, Ignarro LJ. Polymorphisms in endothelial nitric oxide synthase and carotid artery atherosclerosis. J Clin Pathol 2007;60(4):341–4.

144. Tesauro M, Thompson WC, Rogliani P, et al. Intracellular processing of endothelial nitric oxide synthase isoforms associated with differences in severity of cardiopulmonary diseases: cleavage of proteins with aspartate vs. glutamate at position 298. Proc Natl Acad Sci U S A 2000;97(6):2832–5.

145. Persu A, Stoenoiu MS, Messiaen T, et al. Modifier effect of ENOS in autosomal dominant polycystic kidney disease. Hum Mol Genet 2002; 11(3):229–41.

146. Fairchild TA, Fulton D, Fontana JT, et al. Acidic hydrolysis as a mechanism for the cleavage of the Glu(298)->Asp variant of human endothelial nitric-oxide synthase. J Biol Chem 2001;276(28): 26674–9.

147. McDonald DM, Alp NJ, Channon KM. Functional comparison of the endothelial nitric oxide synthase Glu298Asp polymorphic variants in human endothelial cells. Pharmacogenetics 2004;14(12):831–9.

148. Golser R, Gorren AC, Mayer B, et al. Functional characterization of Glu298Asp mutant human endothelial nitric oxide synthase purified from a yeast expression system. Nitric Oxide 2003; 8(1):7–14.

149. Paradossi U, Ciofini E, Clerico A, et al. Endothelial function and carotid intima-media thickness in young healthy subjects among endothelial nitric oxide synthase Glu298->Asp and T-786->C polymorphisms. Stroke 2004;35(6):1305–9.

150. Naber CK, Baumgart D, Altmann C, et al. eNOS 894T allele and coronary blood flow at rest and during adenosine-induced hyperemia. Am J Physiol Heart Circ Physiol 2001;281(5):H1908–12.

151. Philip I, Plantefeve G, Vuillaumier-Barrot S, et al. G894T polymorphism in the endothelial nitric oxide synthase gene is associated with an enhanced vascular responsiveness to phenylephrine. Circulation 1999;99(24):3096–8.

152. Li R, Lyn D, Lapu-Bula R, et al. Relation of endothelial nitric oxide synthase gene to plasma nitric oxide level, endothelial function, and blood pressure in African Americans. Am J Hypertens 2004;17(7):560–7.

153. Rossi GP, Taddei S, Virdis A, et al. The T-786C and Glu298Asp polymorphisms of the endothelial nitric oxide gene affect the forearm blood flow responses of Caucasian hypertensive patients. J Am Coll Cardiol 2003;41(6):938–45.

154. Schmoelzer I, Renner W, Paulweber B, et al. Lack of association of the Glu298Asp polymorphism of endothelial nitric oxide synthase with manifest coronary artery disease, carotid atherosclerosis and forearm vascular reactivity in two Austrian populations. Eur J Clin Invest 2003;33(3):191–8.

155. Lamblin N, Cuilleret FJ, Helbecque N, et al. A common variant of endothelial nitric oxide synthase (Glu298Asp) is associated with collateral development in patients with chronic coronary occlusions. BMC Cardiovasc Disord 2005;5:27.

156. Gulec S, Karabulut H, Ozdemir AO, et al. Glu298Asp polymorphism of the eNOS gene is associated with coronary collateral development. Atherosclerosis 2008;198(2):354–9.

157. Miyamoto Y, Saito Y, Nakayama M, et al. Replication protein A1 reduces transcription of the endothelial nitric oxide synthase gene containing a -786T->C mutation associated with coronary spastic angina. Hum Mol Genet 2000;9(18):2629–37.

158. Cattaruzza M, Guzik TJ, Slodowski W, et al. Shear stress insensitivity of endothelial nitric oxide synthase expression as a genetic risk factor for coronary heart disease. Circ Res 2004;95(8):841–7.

159. Asif AR, Oellerich M, Armstrong VW, et al. T-786C polymorphism of the NOS-3 gene and the endothelial cell response to fluid shear stress-a proteome analysis. J Proteome Res 2009;8(6):3161–8.

160. Wang XL, Sim AS, Wang MX, et al. Genotype dependent and cigarette specific effects on endothelial nitric oxide synthase gene expression and enzyme activity. FEBS Lett 2000;471(1):45–50.

161. Tsukada T, Yokoyama K, Arai T, et al. Evidence of association of the ecNOS gene polymorphism with plasma NO metabolite levels in humans. Biochem Biophys Res Commun 1998;245(1):190–3.

162. Jeerooburkhan N, Jones LC, Bujac S, et al. Genetic and environmental determinants of plasma nitrogen oxides and risk of ischemic heart disease. Hypertension 2001;38(5):1054–61.

163. Yoon Y, Song J, Hong SH, et al. Plasma nitric oxide concentrations and nitric oxide synthase gene polymorphisms in coronary artery disease. Clin Chem 2000;46(10):1626–30.

164. Salimi S, Firoozrai M, Nourmohammadi I, et al. Lack of evidence for contribution of intron4a/b polymorphism of endothelial nitric oxide synthase (NOS3) gene to plasma nitric oxide levels. Acta Cardiol 2008;63(2):229–34.

165. Casas JP, Cavalleri GL, Bautista LE, et al. Endothelial nitric oxide synthase gene polymorphisms and cardiovascular disease: a HuGE review. Am J Epidemiol 2006;164(10):921–35.

166. Vallance P, Chan N. Endothelial function and nitric oxide: clinical relevance. Heart 2001;85(3):342–50.

167. Huang PL. eNOS, metabolic syndrome and cardiovascular disease. Trends Endocrinol Metab 2009;20(6):295–302.

168. Guang-da X, Qiong-shu W, Wen J. A T-786C polymorphism in 5'-flanking region of the endothelial nitric oxide synthase gene and endothelium-dependent arterial dilation in Type 2 diabetes. Diabet Med 2005;22(12):1663–9.

169. Rittig K, Holder K, Stock J, et al. Endothelial NO-synthase intron 4 polymorphism is associated with disturbed in vivo nitric oxide production in individuals prone to type 2 diabetes. Horm Metab Res 2008;40(1):13–7.

170. Sandrim VC, de Syllos RW, Lisboa HR, et al. Influence of eNOS haplotypes on the plasma nitric oxide products concentrations in hypertensive and type 2 diabetes mellitus patients. Nitric Oxide 2007;16(3):348–55.

171. Zintzaras E, Papathanasiou AA, Stefanidis I. Endothelial nitric oxide synthase gene polymorphisms and diabetic nephropathy: a HuGE review and meta-analysis. Genet Med 2009;11(10):695–706.

172. Abhary S, Hewitt AW, Burdon KP, et al. A systematic meta-analysis of genetic association studies for diabetic retinopathy. Diabetes 2009;58(9):2137–47.

173. Odeberg J, Larsson CA, Rastam L, et al. The Asp298 allele of endothelial nitric oxide synthase is a risk factor for myocardial infarction among patients with type 2 diabetes mellitus. BMC Cardiovasc Disord 2008;8:36.

174. Zhang C, Lopez-Ridaura R, Hunter DJ, et al. Common variants of the endothelial nitric oxide synthase gene and the risk of coronary heart disease among U.S. diabetic men. Diabetes 2006;55(7):2140–7.

175. Cai H, Wang X, Colagiuri S, et al. A common Glu298->Asp (894G->T) mutation at exon 7 of the endothelial nitric oxide synthase gene and vascular complications in type 2 diabetes. Diabetes Care 1998;21(12):2195–6.

176. Mollsten A, Lajer M, Jorsal A, et al. The endothelial nitric oxide synthase gene and risk of diabetic nephropathy and development of cardiovascular disease in type 1 diabetes. Mol Genet Metab 2009;97(1):80–4.

177. Bowman BH, Kurosky A. Haptoglobin: the evolutionary product of duplication, unequal crossing over, and point mutation. Adv Hum Genet 1982; 12:189–261, 453–4.

178. Garby L, Noyes WD. Studies on hemoglobin metabolism. I. The kinetic properties of the plasma hemoglobin pool in normal man. J Clin Invest 1959; 38:1479–83.

179. Fagoonee S, Gburek J, Hirsch E, et al. Plasma protein haptoglobin modulates renal iron loading. Am J Pathol 2005;166(4):973–83.

180. Lim SK, Kim H, Lim SK, et al. Increased susceptibility in Hp knockout mice during acute hemolysis. Blood 1998;92(6):1870–7.

181. Kristiansen M, Graversen JH, Jacobsen C, et al. Identification of the haemoglobin scavenger receptor. Nature 2001;409(6817):198–201.

182. Graversen JH, Madsen M, Moestrup SK. CD163: a signal receptor scavenging haptoglobin-hemoglobin complexes from plasma. Int J Biochem Cell Biol 2002;34(4):309–14.

183. Sadrzadeh SM, Graf E, Panter SS, et al. A biologic fenton reagent. J Biol Chem 1984;259(23): 14354–6.

184. Melamed-Frank M, Lache O, Enav BI, et al. Structure-function analysis of the antioxidant properties of haptoglobin. Blood 2001;98(13):3693–8.

185. Miller YI, Altamentova SM, Shaklai N. Oxidation of low-density lipoprotein by hemoglobin stems from a heme-initiated globin radical: antioxidant role of haptoglobin. Biochemistry 1997;36(40): 12189–98.

186. Buehler PW, Abraham B, Vallelian F, et al. Haptoglobin preserves the CD163 hemoglobin scavenger pathway by shielding hemoglobin from peroxidative modification. Blood 2009;113(11):2578–86.

187. Langlois MR, Delanghe JR. Biological and clinical significance of haptoglobin polymorphism in humans. Clin Chem 1996;42(10):1589–600.

188. Levy AP, Hochberg I, Jablonski K, et al. Haptoglobin phenotype is an independent risk factor for cardiovascular disease in individuals with diabetes: the Strong Heart Study. J Am Coll Cardiol 2002;40(11):1984–90.

189. Suleiman M, Aronson D, Asleh R, et al. Haptoglobin polymorphism predicts 30-day mortality and heart failure in patients with diabetes and acute myocardial infarction. Diabetes 2005;54(9):2802–6.

190. Roguin A, Koch W, Kastrati A, et al. Haptoglobin genotype is predictive of major adverse cardiac events in the 1-year period after percutaneous transluminal coronary angioplasty in individuals with diabetes. Diabetes Care 2003; 26(9):2628–31.

191. Costacou T, Ferrell RE, Orchard TJ. Haptoglobin genotype: a determinant of cardiovascular complication risk in type 1 diabetes. Diabetes 2008;57(6): 1702–6.

192. Milman U, Blum S, Shapira C, et al. Vitamin E supplementation reduces cardiovascular events in a subgroup of middle-aged individuals with both type 2 diabetes mellitus and the haptoglobin 2-2 genotype: a prospective double-blinded clinical trial. Arterioscler Thromb Vasc Biol 2008;28(2):341–7.

193. Miller-Lotan R, Miller B, Nakhoul F, et al. Retinal capillary basement membrane thickness in diabetic mice genetically modified at the haptoglobin locus. Diabetes Metab Res Rev 2007;23(2):152–6.

194. Miller-Lotan R, Herskowitz Y, Kalet-Litman S, et al. Increased renal hypertrophy in diabetic mice genetically modified at the haptoglobin locus. Diabetes Metab Res Rev 2005;21(4):332–7.

195. Asleh R, Miller-Lotan R, Aviram M, et al. Haptoglobin genotype is a regulator of reverse cholesterol transport in diabetes in vitro and in vivo. Circ Res 2006;99(12):1419–25.

196. Levy AP, Levy JE, Kalet-Litman S, et al. Haptoglobin genotype is a determinant of iron, lipid peroxidation, and macrophage accumulation in the atherosclerotic plaque. Arterioscler Thromb Vasc Biol 2007;27(1):134–40.

197. De Bacquer D, De Backer G, Langlois M, et al. Haptoglobin polymorphism as a risk factor for coronary heart disease mortality. Atherosclerosis 2001;157(1):161–6.

198. Holme I, Aastveit AH, Hammar N, et al. Haptoglobin and risk of myocardial infarction, stroke, and congestive heart failure in 342,125 men and women in the Apolipoprotein MOrtality RISk study (AMORIS). Ann Med 2009;1–11 [Online].

199. Asleh R, Marsh S, Shilkrut M, et al. Genetically determined heterogeneity in hemoglobin scavenging and susceptibility to diabetic cardiovascular disease. Circ Res 2003;92(11):1193–200.

200. Asleh R, Guetta J, Kalet-Litman S, et al. Haptoglobin genotype- and diabetes-dependent differences in iron-mediated oxidative stress in vitro and in vivo. Circ Res 2005;96(4):435–41.

201. Kalet-Litman S, Moreno PR, Levy AP. The haptoglobin 2-2 genotype is associated with increased redox active hemoglobin derived iron in the atherosclerotic plaque. Atherosclerosis 2010; 209(1):28–31.

202. Levy AP, Purushothaman KR, Levy NS, et al. Downregulation of the hemoglobin scavenger receptor in individuals with diabetes and the Hp 2-2 genotype: implications for the response to intraplaque hemorrhage and plaque vulnerability. Circ Res 2007; 101(1):106–10.

203. Timmermann M, Hogger P. Oxidative stress and 8-iso-prostaglandin F(2alpha) induce ectodomain shedding of CD163 and release of tumor necrosis factor-alpha from human monocytes. Free Radic Biol Med 2005;39(1): 98–107.

204. Boyle JJ, Harrington HA, Piper E, et al. Coronary intraplaque hemorrhage evokes a novel atheroprotective macrophage phenotype. Am J Pathol 2009;174(3):1097–108.

205. Asleh R, Blum S, Kalet-Litman S, et al. Correction of HDL dysfunction in individuals with diabetes and the haptoglobin 2-2 genotype. Diabetes 2008; 57(10):2794–800.

206. Farbstein D, Levy AP. Pharmacogenomics and the prevention of vascular complications in diabetes mellitus. Therapy 2009;6(4):531–8.

207. Levy AP, Asleh R, Blum S, et al. Haptoglobin: basic and clinical aspects. Antioxid Redox Signal 2010; 12(2):293–304.

Influence of Glycemic Control on the Development of Diabetic Cardiovascular and Kidney Disease

Sandeep A. Saha, MD[a,b,*], Katherine R. Tuttle, MD[a,b]

KEYWORDS

- CKD • Heart disease • Metformin • Sulfonylureas
- Thiazolidinediones • Insulin • Incretin • PKC inhibitors

The global prevalence of diabetes mellitus (DM) continues to increase; the World Health Organization estimates that more than 180 million people worldwide have diabetes, and this number is projected to reach a staggering 366 million by 2030.[1,2] In addition, the proportion of diabetic patients older than 65 years is estimated to increase by 134% by 2030. Diabetes leads to the development of a host of micro- and macrovascular complications, which collectively lead to substantial morbidity and mortality. Among the microvascular complications of diabetes, diabetic kidney disease (DKD) is the most common, affecting approximately 30% of those with type 1 DM and up to 40% of those with type 2 DM.[3] Macrovascular complications from diabetes cause a 2- to 4-fold increase in the incidence of cardiovascular disease (CVD) and up to twice the mortality from cardiovascular causes as compared with nondiabetic individuals.[4] CVD affects about 14% of persons with type 1 DM[5] and up to 40% of those with type 2 DM.[6] DKD is one of the most important risk amplifiers for CVD;[7] indeed, the rate of mortality (predominantly due to CVD causes) in type 2 DM approaches 20% per year when kidney function

measurably declines.[8] By 2025, the world is estimated to spend more than US$ 302.5 billion in the prevention and treatment of DM.[9]

The significance of glycemic control in the prevention of DKD and diabetic CVD has come under increased scrutiny, especially since the recent publication of some large randomized clinical trials in this field. Although there is a great deal of overlap between the occurrence of CVD and chronic kidney disease (CKD) in patients with diabetes, intensive glycemic control has led to disparate effects on the occurrence of micro- and macrovascular complications in large randomized trials. This observation may be ascribed to the fact that, in addition to hyperglycemia, several traditional (such as hypertension and dyslipidemia) as well as nontraditional risk factors (such as insulin resistance and advanced glycation end products) also affect the occurrence of vascular complications in diabetes. Many drug classes and insulin regimens have been used to effect glycemic control (variably defined using either plasma glucose levels or glycosylated hemoglobin [HbA_{1c}] levels) in large randomized clinical trials in various patient populations. Finally, differences

Financial disclosures: S.A. Saha, none; K.R. Tuttle, none.

[a] Providence Medical Research Center and Providence Sacred Heart Medical Center, 104 West 5th Avenue, Suite 350E, Spokane, WA 99204, USA

[b] Department of Medicine, University of Washington School of Medicine, Box 356420, Seattle, WA 98195-6420, USA

* Corresponding author. Providence Medical Research Center and Providence Sacred Heart Medical Center, 104 West 5th Avenue, Suite 350E, Spokane, WA 99204.

E-mail address: sahas@uw.edu

Cardiol Clin 28 (2010) 497–516
doi:10.1016/j.ccl.2010.04.008
0733-8651/10/$ – see front matter © 2010 Elsevier Inc. All rights reserved.

in the trial design, size, event rates (and therefore statistical power), duration of follow-up, and the level of glycemic control achieved in the comparator group further confound interpretation and application of the results from large randomized controlled trials. In this article, the authors review the current clinical evidence linking glycemic control using various classes of antihyperglycemic agents to the occurrence of DKD and diabetic CVD and provide the reader with recommendations for the application of the current evidence to the care of the individual patient.

INDIVIDUAL DRUG CLASSES
Metformin and Other Biguanides

Metformin is a biguanide that has been used as a glucose-lowering drug for many years. Metformin continues to be the first-line oral antihyperglycemic agent for the treatment of the majority of patients with type 2 DM. The hypoglycemic effect is ascribed to its ability to reduce hepatic glucose output by inhibition of glycogenolysis, as well as improved insulin sensitivity in the peripheral tissues, especially skeletal muscle.[10] Earlier studies, including the University Group Diabetes Program (UGDP) study, showed that the biguanide phenformin was associated with increased cardiovascular mortality and increased all-cause mortality (which also included 1 lactic acidosis–associated death) when compared with the combination of insulin and placebo allocations.[11] Although there is continued concern about the risk of lactic acidosis with metformin use, actual incidence is estimated at about 0.03 cases per 1000 patient-years, which is about 10- to 20-fold lower than the risk with phenformin.[12] However, when lactic acidosis does occur, the death rate is approximately 50%.[13,14] Patients with CKD are at an increased risk of lactic acidosis, and consequently, patients with decreased kidney function should not be treated with metformin. The US Food and Drug Administration (FDA) has determined that the drug is contraindicated based on serum creatinine levels greater than 1.5 mg/dL in men or greater than 1.4 mg/dL in women. Notably, the FDA labeling has not been updated to reflect estimated glomerular filtration rate (eGFR), the current standard for kidney function assessment.[15] Advantages of metformin use include the absence of weight gain, reduction in plasma insulin levels, low incidence of hypoglycemia and other adverse effects, and low cost of therapy.

The United Kingdom Prospective Diabetes Study (UKPDS) 34 was a randomized controlled trial performed in 15 medical centers in the United Kingdom in the 1980s and is the largest and longest clinical trial that studied the use of metformin in patients with newly diagnosed type 2 DM.[16] A total of 753 overweight persons (>120% of ideal body weight) were randomized to conventional therapy, which included predominantly dietary modification along with various glucose-lowering medications as needed (n = 411), or to metformin in escalating doses, with the target to achieve near-normal glycemia (up to 2250 mg/d, n = 342), and followed up for a median duration of 10.7 years. A secondary analysis also compared the effects of intensive glucose-lowering therapy in these 342 patients randomized to metformin with those randomized to chlorpropamide (n = 265), glibenclamide (n = 277), and insulin (n = 409). Weight gain was least with metformin use and comparable with that seen in the conventional therapy group, while plasma insulin levels were also lowest in the metformin group and persisted throughout the study period. Fasting plasma glucose (FPG) and HbA_{1c} levels showed a marked decrease in the first year after initiation of metformin but subsequently increased slowly to approach those in the conventional therapy group by about 10 years postrandomization. When compared with conventional therapy, metformin use significantly reduced the risk of diabetes-related adverse events by 32% and all-cause mortality by 36%, and both these risk reductions were significantly greater than those seen with the use of sulfonylureas (SUs) or insulin. Metformin also significantly reduced the risk of diabetes-related deaths and myocardial infarctions (MIs) when compared with conventional therapy, with no significant differences when compared with SUs or insulin. No cases of fatal lactic acidosis were seen with metformin use in this study. In another analysis from the UKPDS cohort, 537 patients with uncontrolled type 2 DM in spite of maximal SU therapy were randomized either to continuation of the same therapy (n = 269) or to addition of metformin to the existing regimen (n = 268) and followed up for a median of 6.6 years thereafter. This group of patients was older, had a greater degree of hyperglycemia, and was less overweight than the patients enlisted in the earlier study. The effects of metformin on FPG and HbA_{1c} levels were similar to those seen in the larger study, and no significant changes in body weight or plasma insulin levels were seen after addition of metformin. Unexpectedly, the addition of metformin to SU therapy caused a 96% increase in the risk of diabetes-related death and a 60% increase in the risk of all-cause mortality in these patients, but no significant changes were seen in the risk of MI, stroke, or microvascular complications. Although the reasons for the unexpected results in the latter analysis are not known, the investigators concluded that metformin may be used as a first-line pharmacologic therapy in diet-treated overweight patients with type 2 DM.

When metformin was initially approved for clinical use by the FDA, it was contraindicated in patients with decreased kidney function and in situations such as hypoxemia, liver dysfunction, and during the use of radiocontrast dye.[17] Subsequently, based on findings that many cases of lactic acidosis were seen in those with heart failure,[18] the use of metformin was additionally contraindicated in patients with heart failure necessitating medical therapy. However, metformin use may be safe in patients with early-stage CKD (no decrease in eGFR), congestive heart failure (CHF) without acute decompensation, or chronic obstructive pulmonary disease (COPD). In an open-label, prospective randomized trial, 393 patients with type 2 DM (which included 94 patients with CHF and 91 with COPD) who were already on metformin therapy were randomized either to continue metformin or to discontinue its use and followed up for about 4 years. The incidence of micro-and macrovascular events (which included cardiovascular and total mortality) was identical in both groups, and the group that discontinued metformin had significantly greater weight gain and higher HbA_{1c} levels.[19] Conversely, in a retrospective cohort of 1833 patients with incident heart failure who were prescribed metformin and/or SU therapy for type 2 DM, the use of metformin alone or in combination with SU was associated with reduced mortality or hospitalization when compared with SU monotherapy.[20] A retrospective cohort study of 24,953 Medicare beneficiaries with type 2 DM discharged after an acute MI showed that the use of metformin along with a thiazolidinedione (TZD) significantly reduced mortality in the first year, with similar results among patients with CHF.[21]

The Comparative Outcomes Study of Metformin Intervention versus Conventional (COSMIC) Approach was a postmarketing safety surveillance study with a randomized, open-label, active-comparator, parallel-group trial design, performed in type 2 diabetic patients who were suboptimally controlled on diet or SU alone.[22] Patients were randomized to 2 primary treatment groups, metformin (n = 7227) and usual care (n = 1505), and within the primary treatment groups, patients received either monotherapy or combination therapy based on their prior treatment regimen. The primary study objective was to compare the incidence of serious adverse events, death, and hospitalization. After 12 months, the incidence of serious adverse events was similar in both primary

treatment groups, and the risks of all-cause mortality and hospitalizations were also similar between the groups. Mean plasma lactate levels were also similar in both primary treatment groups, and no cases of lactic acidosis were observed. However, this trial excluded patients with later-stage CKD (serum creatinine level>1.5 mg/dL in men or >1.4 mg/dL in women) and only enrolled patients with "acceptable health" status. To evaluate the feasibility of using metformin in patients with type 2 DM and heart failure, researchers from Canada designed the Patients with Heart Failure and Type 2 Diabetes Treated with Placebo or Metformin (PHANTOM) study, a multicenter, prospective, randomized, blinded, placebo-controlled pilot study designed to examine functionality, morbidity, and mortality outcomes during a 6-month period. Patients would be eligible for inclusion if they had physician-diagnosed heart failure (New York Heart Association [NYHA] class II or worse) and type 2 DM and were on less than 1500 mg of metformin daily. Despite a contraindication to its use, the researchers found that metformin was the most commonly prescribed oral antidiabetic agent (51% of the first 58 patients screened) and was prescribed in combination with insulin more than any other oral agent.[23] Observational data in Canada, Europe, and the United States have shown that 20% to 25% of patients receiving metformin therapy also have concomitant heart failure, and the use of metformin in patients with heart failure has increased by more than 50% in the United States in recent years.[24] The PHANTOM study was eventually abandoned amidst issues of low enrollment and questions about its impact on mainstream clinical practice. At present, the presence of heart failure is no longer a contraindication to the use of metformin, although caution is still advised in patients with conditions in which there is significant tissue hypoperfusion and hypoxemia, including decompensated CHF.[25]

Sulfonylureas and Meglitinides

SUs are a class of insulin secretagogues, which bind to the SU receptor (SUR), a subunit of the ATP-dependent potassium (K_{ATP}) channels present on the surface of all mammalian cells. The resultant inhibition of potassium release through these K_{ATP} channels in the pancreatic islet beta cells causes membrane depolarization, which in turn activates calcium channels causing increased calcium influx into the cells, which consequently stimulates the release of insulin. In the UGDP study, the use of tolbutamide, an older SU, was found to be associated with a significant increase in cardiac mortality, which led to the premature (and controversial) termination of the tolbutamide arm of this study.[26] Subsequent studies showed that the older SUs may adversely affect ischemic preconditioning of myocardium in the hearts of diabetic patients,[27] thereby decreasing the extent of myocardial salvage through reperfusion therapies after an acute MI. A new subtype of the SUR (SUR2) was subsequently cloned, which is selectively expressed in skeletal and cardiac muscle, and this SUR subtype was thought to be associated with the potential cardiotoxicity of the older SUs.[28] Newer SUs, such as glimepiride, gliclazide, and metaglinides such as repaglinide, preferentially bind to the SUR1 receptor on pancreatic islet beta cells and have been shown to stimulate insulin secretion but to not block ischemic preconditioning of myocardium in animal models[29–31] and in clinical studies.[32]

In the UKPDS 33 study,[33] 3867 patients with newly diagnosed type 2 DM were randomized to conventional glycemic control, which included dietary modification and subsequent addition of medications for symptomatic hyperglycemia for an FPG level of more than 15 mmol/L (n = 1138), or to intensive glycemic control with a target of 6 mmol/L or less (near-normal glycemia) using either SUs (n = 1573) or insulin (n = 1156). Three different SUs were used in this study: chlorpropamide (n = 788), glibenclamide (n = 615), and glipizide (n = 170). Of the patients randomized to conventional therapy, 702 needed addition of antidiabetic medications; 370 of these patients were given SUs. The primary study end points were any diabetes-related event, diabetes-related death, and all-cause mortality; several clinical end points as well as surrogate markers of micro- and macrovascular disease were also defined and recorded. All 3 SUs caused an initial drop in FPG and HbA$_{1c}$ levels in the first year, but these levels subsequently started to slowly increase through the rest of the study period. However, the median HbA$_{1c}$ levels during 10 years in the intensive treatment group were about 0.9 percentage points lower than that in the conventional group (a reduction of approximately 11%), with chlorpropamide causing the greatest (median HbA$_{1c}$, 6.7%) median reduction, followed by insulin (7.1%) and glibenclamide (7.2%). Intensive treatment led to a significant decrease in diabetes-related events (mean relative risk reduction [RRR], 12%, P = .009), but no significant differences in diabetes-related death or all-cause mortality were observed when compared with conventional treatment. Patients who received intensive treatment recorded a significant 25% RRR in microvascular

complications (P = .0099) when compared with conventional treatment, with the majority of this effect attributed to reduction in the need for retinal photocoagulation (mean RRR, 29%, P = .0031). The risks of development of kidney failure, as well as of deaths from CKD, were not significantly affected, although the event rates were rather small in this study. The incidences of microalbuminuria, overt proteinuria, or doubling of serum creatinine levels were also not affected by the use of intensive treatment at the end of 15 years. With regard to macrovascular complications, the effect of intensive treatment on MI was modest (mean RRR, 16%, P = .052), with no significant effect on stroke, heart failure, or sudden death. No significant differences in clinical outcomes were seen among the 3 SUs used in this study, although significantly higher systolic and diastolic pressures were noted among patients receiving chlorpropamide. A significantly greater proportion of patients in the intensive treatment had hypoglycemia throughout the study duration (P<.0001), with the highest being among those randomized to insulin therapy. Weight gain was also significantly greater in the intensive treatment group (mean difference in weight, 3.1 kg at 10 years, P<.0001), and the weight gain was significantly higher with insulin use as compared with SU use. However, the UKPDS results did not show any evidence of increased cardiovascular events with the use of SUs, as suggested by the UGDP study with tolbutamide. The investigators concluded that the extent of glycemic control, rather than the pharmacologic agent used, primarily dictated the magnitude of benefit, especially in microvascular events, in patients with newly diagnosed type 2 DM.

The efficacy of glycemic control with SUs tends to wane over time, and this tendency is largely attributed to the progression of type 2 DM itself rather than the exhaustion of pancreatic beta cell function caused by the secretagogue action of SUs. A Diabetes Outcome Progression Trial (ADOPT) evaluated the durability of glycemic control using rosiglitazone, metformin, and glyburide as initial monotherapy in a randomized, double-blind controlled trial involving 4360 patients with recently diagnosed type 2 DM.[34] The cumulative incidence of monotherapy failure at the end of 5 years was highest with glyburide (34%) as compared with metformin (21%) and rosiglitazone (15%). Of the 3 agents used, glyburide caused the greatest initial decrease in FPG and HbA$_{1c}$ levels at 6 months, but subsequently values of both these glycemic measures increased the most with glyburide, with annual increases of 5.6 mg/dL in FPG level and 0.24% in HbA$_{1c}$ level.

Beta cell function was increased by all 3 agents used and was significantly greater with the use of glyburide at 6 months (in keeping with its mechanism of action) but subsequently declined in all 3 groups, with the greatest rate of decline in the glyburide group. However, at the end of 5 years, beta cell function in the glyburide group was similar to that in the rosiglitazone group and was lowest in the metformin group. SUs tend to cause hypoglycemia more than other classes of oral agents and are associated with weight gain (to a smaller extent than rosiglitazone), and these adverse effects may worsen cardiac vulnerability to ischemia and arrhythmias and also contribute to peripheral insulin resistance. There is epidemiologic data that suggest increased risk of death with higher doses of first-generation SUs,[35] and although these agents have not been adequately studied in high-risk situations such as hypoxia or acute MI, it is prudent to withdraw use of first-generation SUs after an acute MI.

Meglitinides are a new class of insulin secretagogues, which preferentially bind to a specific domain on the SUR1 receptor on the pancreatic islet beta cells, and 2 analogs, repaglinide and nateglinide, are currently available for clinical use. A Cochrane review that included 3781 patients enrolled in 15 parallel randomized controlled trials showed that repaglinide reduced HbA_{1c} levels at 16 weeks to a greater extent than nateglinide, and although the cumulative clinical experience and data on adverse events with these agents are limited, these drugs are generally well tolerated.[36] Repaglinide is at least as effective in reducing HbA_{1c} and FPG levels as SUs, metformin, or TZDs and is also effective in combination therapy with other oral antidiabetic agents.[37] Some studies show a better effect of repaglinide on postprandial hyperglycemia—it enhances the early phase insulin release after a meal, but having a short duration of action necessitates its administration before each meal. Its propensity to induce hypoglycemia is similar to that of SUs, and repaglinide is associated with less weight gain than SUs or TZDs. Repaglinide may be particularly useful in the treatment of type 2 DM when metformin use is contraindicated, when there is a need for flexible dosing (such as in the elderly), or when postprandial hyperglycemia needs to be specifically addressed. Repaglinide is safe and effective in patients with type 2 DM complicated by low eGFR and may be an appropriate treatment choice, even in individuals with advanced CKD.[38,39] However, no published studies have investigated the effects of repaglinide on hard clinical outcomes (cardiovascular or renal), including mortality, although several studies indicate

beneficial effects on cardiovascular surrogate end points, such as carotid intima-media thickness, inflammatory markers, lipid parameters, and oxidative stress.[37] In addition, little data are available on the potential cardiotoxicity of these agents, although their short duration of action, binding on a domain on the SU receptor distinct from other SUs, and greater affinity for the pancreatic K_{ATP} channels suggest that this risk is probably lower than that of the older SUs.

Thiazolidinediones

TZDs are a newer class of oral antidiabetic drugs that act primarily as insulin sensitizing agents by binding to and stimulating the peroxisome proliferator-activated receptor (PPAR) γ, an isoform of the PPAR family of nuclear receptors that regulate expression of genes involved in many metabolic processes, including glucose homeostasis, adipogenesis, and lipid metabolism.[40,41] Their antihyperglycemic effect is ascribed to increased peripheral glucose uptake in skeletal muscle and adipose tissue and reduction in hepatic glucose output. However, TZDs have been shown to have several pleiotropic effects, including antioxidant, antiinflammatory, antiproliferative and antifibrotic effects, on the blood vessel wall and glomeruli,[42] and pioglitazone has been shown to favorably affect systolic blood pressure and lipid parameters in patients with type 2 DM.[43]

In contrast to metformin and SUs, clinical studies of TZDs have focused on their effects on macrovascular outcomes, whereas no clinical studies in humans have examined their effect on microvascular clinical end points, including renal outcomes, to date. Animal studies have shown direct salutary effects of TZDs on urinary protein excretion and development of overt nephropathy, effects that seem to be independent of the glycemic effect but associated with blood pressure reduction. Human studies have shown that currently available TZDs significantly, consistently, and independently of their glycemic effect reduce urinary albumin excretion (UAE), the most commonly used biomarker for kidney damage.[44–50] However, tight blood pressure control is considered to be even more important than glycemic control in reducing UAE and protecting against DKD progression in patients with type 2 DM, and whether TZDs can reduce UAE independent of blood pressure–lowering effects still remains unclear.[42] Some cases of new or worsening diabetic macular edema have been seen with rosiglitazone,[51] and the product labels for rosiglitazone and pioglitazone have been appropriately modified pending more studies.[52,53] In the absence of large randomized clinical trials specifically designed to study effects of TZDs on hard clinical outcomes of microvascular disease, these medications should be used primarily for their glucose-lowering effects in patients with type 2 DM.

Many studies have shown that TZDs cause reduction of atherosclerotic burden by reduction of progression of carotid intima-media thickness when compared with placebo or active comparators[54–56] and that TZDs also reduce neointimal hyperplasia after coronary stent implantation as measured by intravascular ultrasound in patients with type 2 DM.[57] In a meta-analysis of 7 prospective randomized trials involving a total of 608 patients, TZDs have been shown to reduce the risk of repeat revascularization after percutaneous coronary intervention.[58] These results, along with the numerous animal and preclinical human studies that show that TZDs have many pleiotropic beneficial effects on progression of atherosclerosis and endothelial dysfunction, suggested that TZDs may significantly reduce adverse cardiovascular events in patients with type 2 DM, and several clinical trials were performed to evaluate this premise. Although numerous studies have been performed using rosiglitazone, many of them were designed to study its effect primarily on glycemic control, and the 2 largest trials using rosiglitazone were performed in nondiabetic patients[59] or patients with newly diagnosed type 2 DM.[34] In 2007, a controversial meta-analysis[60] of 42 randomized trials using rosiglitazone as well as a retrospective analysis of a large health care utilization database[61] showed that rosiglitazone use was associated with an approximately 40% increased risk of MI when compared with non-TZD use, and this spurred a deluge of repeat analyses[62–65] and similar analyses with pioglitazone,[66–68] critical commentaries about the studies themselves and the methods used in the various meta-analyses,[69,70] and even the FDA approval process.[71] Since then, the role of TZDs in the prevention of diabetic macrovascular complications has been plagued by controversy and uncertainty.

To date, the largest randomized controlled clinical trial that evaluated the use of TZD (pioglitazone) for prevention of macrovascular clinical events in patients with type 2 DM is the PROactive (Prospective Pioglitazone Clinical Trial in Macrovascular Events) trial,[43] which enrolled 5238 patients with type 2 DM with clinical evidence of macrovascular disease and randomized them to increasing doses of pioglitazone (15–45 mg/d, n = 2605) or matching placebo (n = 2633) in addition to their preexisting medications. All participants were kept on optimal medical therapy based on established guidelines[72] during the study period, which included antiplatelet, antihypertensive, and antidyslipidemic agents, and followed up for a mean of 34.5 months. About 46% of these patients had a history of prior MI, about 42% had evidence of microvascular disease, and nearly 50% had 2 or more macrovascular disease criteria, making this a group of patients with high baseline cardiovascular risk. Patients with planned revascularization procedures, those with CHF (NYHA class II or worse), and those on hemodialysis were excluded. The primary end point was a composite of all-cause mortality, nonfatal MI, stroke, acute coronary syndrome, endovascular or surgical intervention in the coronary or leg arteries, and above-knee amputations. The main secondary end point was also a composite of all-cause mortality, nonfatal MI and stroke, as well as individual components of the primary composite end point. Of note is the fact that CHF (necessitating hospitalization) or CHF-related death were not part of the primary study end point and therefore was not centrally adjudicated. Pioglitazone had a nonsignificant RRR of 10% on the primary composite end point ($P = .095$) but significantly reduced the risk of the main secondary end point (mean relative risk [RR], 0.84, $P = .027$), and the latter effect persisted even after adjustment for several established cardiovascular risk factors. The Kaplan-Meier curves for the primary end point showed a tendency toward increased adverse events in the pioglitazone arm in the first 12 to 14 months, after which the curves crossed and slowly diverged until study end but did not reach statistical significance. For the main secondary end point, the Kaplan-Meier curves did not start separating until about 12 to 14 months or so and did show statistical significance at study end. There was no significant effect of pioglitazone use on any of the individual clinical outcomes measured in the study. Pioglitazone was also associated with small, but statistically significant, improvements in the levels of triglycerides and high-density lipoprotein (HDL) cholesterol and in the low-density lipoprotein (LDL) cholesterol/HDL cholesterol ratio. In addition, systolic blood pressure levels were slightly but significantly lowered by pioglitazone in this study, and although hard clinical outcomes for microvascular events were not recorded, changes in UAE were similar in both treatment groups. The use of metformin and insulin were significantly increased in the placebo group during the study, and although changes in the use of other medications were not significantly different, loop diuretics were prescribed more often (7.7%) in the pioglitazone group as compared with placebo (5.4%). The mean absolute decrease in HbA$_{1c}$ level with pioglitazone use was a modest 0.5% when compared with placebo, and the use of statins was increased by about 12.4% as compared with baseline (which was low at 43%). Reported cases of heart failure, as well as serious heart failure necessitating hospitalization, were significantly more in the pioglitazone group, and more patients who were prescribed pioglitazone had clinical evidence of edema without heart failure (562 vs 341 in placebo group). However, cases of fatal heart failure (centrally adjudicated) did not differ between the 2 groups, although the event rates were rather small (25 vs 22 in placebo group). In addition, the risk of symptomatic hypoglycemia was also significantly higher with pioglitazone (28% vs 20% with placebo, $P<.0001$), and the pioglitazone group has significantly greater weight gain (mean increase of 3.6 kg vs a mean loss of 0.4 kg in placebo group, $P<.0001$). A subgroup analysis of the PROactive trial participants with a history of prior MI 6 months or more before study enrollment (n = 2445; 1230 randomized to pioglitazone and 1215 randomized to placebo), followed up for a mean of 2.85 years, showed that pioglitazone caused a significant 28% mean risk reduction in the prespecified end point of fatal and nonfatal MI and a 19% mean RR in the cardiac composite end point of nonfatal MI, coronary revascularization, acute coronary syndrome (ACS), and cardiac death.[73] However, in this prespecified and post hoc subgroup analysis, the incidence of the main secondary composite end point of the PROactive study tended to be lower with pioglitazone (12% vs 14.7% in placebo group, $P = .0585$) and the main primary composite end point was not significantly affected (21.4% vs 24%, $P = .1351$). No significant benefit of pioglitazone was seen for any of the individual cardiovascular study end points except the risk of ACS (estimated hazard ratio [HR], 0.63, $P = .0346$). In this analysis too, the incidence of heart failure and heart failure necessitating hospitalization were significantly higher with pioglitazone (estimated HR, 1.43 and 1.45, respectively), but fatal heart failure did not differ between the 2 groups. Statin use improved substantially during the course of this study in both groups (from 51% at baseline to 63% at study end), and again, more patients in the pioglitazone group were prescribed loop diuretics than those in the placebo group. The salutary effects of pioglitazone on triglyceride and HDL cholesterol levels and on LDL cholesterol/HDL cholesterol ratio were also seen in this subgroup, but blood pressure was largely unchanged with the use of pioglitazone in this subgroup. The mean absolute decrease in HbA$_{1c}$ level with the use of pioglitazone was 0.4%. In the main PROactive study and the latter subgroup analysis, pioglitazone use was associated with modest decreases in HbA$_{1c}$ levels and small improvements in the lipid profiles, and, in the case of the main trial, in systolic blood pressure; the trial participants had overall improved use of statins. Clinical trials that preceded PROactive essentially showed that in patients with type 2 DM, greater success is achieved in reducing adverse cardiovascular events by optimizing control of blood pressure and level of lipids than with control of glycemia per se. The effect of pioglitazone on cardiovascular events in the PROactive study are at best modest and may be the cumulative result of the overall improvements in the metabolic profile of its participants. However, among high-risk patients with type 2 DM, including those with a history of prior MI, pioglitazone did not increase all-cause or cardiac mortality but did increase the risk of heart failure, as well as hospitalization for heart failure, by about 40%. An ongoing trial called the Pioglitazone Protects DM Patients Against Re-Infarction Study (NCT00212004) is currently underway and aims to enroll 3000 patients with type 2 DM and prior MI and randomize them to pioglitazone or usual care, including diet, weight reduction, exercise, and/or SU therapy. The primary study end points are cardiovascular mortality and hospitalization for cardiovascular events, and patients will be followed up for at least 2 years.[74]

Recently, 2 important additions to the rosiglitazone literature have been published. In response to the meta-analyses published in 2007, which suggested that the use of rosiglitazone tended to increase cardiac mortality and substantially increase the risk for MI by about 40%,[60,62] the manufacturers of rosiglitazone, GlaxoSmithKline (King of Prussia, PA, USA), performed a patient-level analysis involving a total of 14,237 subjects with type 2 DM from 42 GSK-sponsored double-blind, controlled studies and reported that the HR for MI with the use of rosiglitazone using data pooled from the aforementioned studies was 1.30 (95% confidence interval [CI], 1.004–1.69).[75] Although event rates were small for each of the comparisons made using exact logistic regression models and the risk estimates had wide confidence intervals invariably including unity, the investigators reported that the incidence of CHF may be higher when rosiglitazone is combined with SUs or insulin. A retrospective cohort study was performed using insurance claims data over a 7-year period to assess the risk of MI and coronary revascularization in patients with type 2 DM who were started on rosiglitazone (n $\approx$ 57,000), pioglitazone (n $\approx$ 51,000), metformin (n ≈ 275,000), or SUs (n ≈ 160,000). This study showed that in the absence of insulin, TZD-containing treatment regimens tended to have lower risk of MI and coronary revascularization than regimens containing SUs but higher risk than regimens containing metformin. Head-to-head comparisons showed that rosiglitazone was associated with a nonsignificant 21% increase for MI during on-treatment time as compared with pioglitazone.[76] This study was also performed by GSK.

The RECORD (Rosiglitazone Evaluated for Cardiac Outcomes and Regulation of Glycaemia in Diabetes) trial was a multicenter, open-label clinical trial (funded by GSK), which included 4447 patients with type 2 DM suboptimally controlled on metformin or SUs and randomly assigned to addition to rosiglitazone (n = 2220) or to a combination of SU and metformin (n = 2227).[77] The overall primary event rate was lower than anticipated, thereby reducing the statistical power of the study. After a mean follow-up of 5.5 years, the incidence of the primary study outcome (cardiovascular hospitalization or cardiovascular death) was nearly identical in both groups, yielding a HR of 0.99 and meeting criteria for noninferiority. No significant changes in mortality, MI, or stroke were seen between the 2 treatment groups. However, heart failure causing hospitalization or death was significantly more in the rosiglitazone group (HR, 2.10, P = .001). Fatal heart failure was also higher with the use of rosiglitazone (10 vs 2 cases in the active-comparator group). A prespecified subgroup analysis stratified patients based on presence or absence of prior ischemic heart disease and found that more primary events tended to occur with rosiglitazone use among those with prior ischemic heart disease. The addition of rosiglitazone was associated with a significant mean weight gain of 3.8 to 4.1 kg. Significant beneficial effects were seen on LDL cholesterol and HDL cholesterol levels with the addition of rosiglitazone when compared with baseline values, but this observation may partly be attributable to the fact that statin use (from about 19% to about 50%) and fibrate use (from 5.5% to about 11%) increased considerably during the trial period. In addition, the risk of fractures (including the spine and upper and distal lower limb) was higher in those randomized to rosiglitazone, mainly in women (overall RR, 1.57; RR in women, 1.82), a finding that was suggested previously in the ADOPT trial. Also, a possible increase in "nonserious" cases of macular edema was seen among patients randomized to rosiglitazone. No data are available on the effect of rosiglitazone on renal outcomes or surrogate markers of kidney damage. The overall risk of malignancy did not differ between the 2 groups.

The effect of TZDs on macrovascular events in patients with type 2 DM is still unclear. Interpretation of data from large randomized trials to evaluate the effect of glycemic control with TZDs on clinical outcomes has been confounded by low event rates, short follow-up durations, pleiotropic effects of TZDs on blood pressure and lipid parameters, and improved medical management of other cardiovascular risk factors during the trial period. Among high-risk patients with type 2 DM and evidence of macrovascular disease, pioglitazone may modestly reduce the risk of major cardiovascular events, but whether this is due to direct effects of the drug itself or due to its pleiotropic effects on lipid metabolism and possibly blood pressure is still undetermined. Both pioglitazone and rosiglitazone significantly increase the risk of heart failure and peripheral edema and are associated with significant weight gain. Data regarding their effect on microvascular outcomes are scarce in the large clinical trials, and there is suggestion of increase in the risk of macular edema with these agents. Questions about the possibility of increased risk of MI with rosiglitazone in comparison with other oral agents including pioglitazone still remain, pending further clinical investigation and experience with the use of these agents.

Insulin

The use of insulin is an important component of the treatment for type 1 DM, as well as for patients with type 2 DM in whom glycemic control remains or becomes suboptimal with the use of oral antidiabetic agents. The DCCT (Diabetes Control and Complications Trial) studied 1441 patients with type 1 DM with no CVD at baseline, who were randomized to intensive or to conventional glycemic control, for a mean duration of 6.5 years. At the end of the study period, the mean HbA_{1c} level in the intensive group was 7.4%, whereas that in the conventional group was 9.1%. Intensive treatment in DCCT significantly decreased the risk of albuminuria by 39% and the risk of neuropathy by 60% when compared with conventional treatment. Although the risk of macrovascular events was also reduced by 41%, this was not statistically significant.[78] The DCCT/EDIC (Epidemiology of Diabetes Interventions and Complications) study followed up 93% of individuals in the original DCCT cohort for a mean of 17 years since randomization and found that in those who were originally assigned to intensive treatment during the DCCT, the risk of macrovascular events was significantly reduced by 42%, and the risk of serious CVD events was also significantly reduced by 57% (P = .02 for both).[79] In a combined cohort of 1602 individuals with type 1 DM enrolled in the DCCT/EDIC and the Pittsburgh Epidemiology of Diabetes Complications studies, intensive treatment was associated with approximately 50% reduction in the risk of microvascular disease (proliferative retinopathy, nephropathy) and approximately 36% reduction in the risk of cardiovascular events.[5]

Among patients with type 2 DM, several epidemiologic studies have shown a correlation between glycemic control and risk of CVD, and for every 1% increase in HbA_{1c} level more than 7%, coronary heart disease events increased by 40% and mortality by 26%.[80] Although the use of insulin in patients with type 2 DM has been historically hindered by concerns about weight gain and risk of hypoglycemia, newer evidence has shown that insulin has a host of antiinflammatory and potentially cardioprotective effects.[81] This is coupled by the fact that in most patients with type 2 DM of long duration, the efficacy of oral antidiabetic agents to maintain adequate glycemic control wanes over time, necessitating either the addition of insulin to their treatment regimen or, in some cases, switching their treatment to insulin monotherapy. Clinical trials studying the use of insulin in various settings have produced disparate results. The landmark UKPDS 33 randomized 3867 newly diagnosed patients with type 2 DM who had failed a 3-month dietary modification trial to intensive therapy using SU or insulin with a target FPG level of 6 mmol/L or less or to conventional therapy with diet. After 10 years, intensive treatment lowered the HbA_{1c} level to 7% (as compared with 7.9% with conventional treatment) and led to a 25% risk reduction in microvascular events, mostly because of reduction in the need for retinal photocoagulation.[33] An observational follow-up of 3277 patients enrolled in UKPDS up to 10 years postrandomization showed that the achieved differences in HbA_{1c} levels during the trial period were lost in the first year after study completion. However, in the patients originally randomized to the intensive treatment group, the RRRs in microvascular events persisted (24%), and in addition, significant risk reduction in all-cause mortality (13%) and MI (15%) were observed.[6] The Euro Heart Survey on Diabetes and the Heart studied 4676 patients with coronary artery disease (CAD), of whom 1425 had previously diagnosed DM and 452 were newly diagnosed with DM. Among the 378 patients with known DM who were treated with insulin, the adjusted risk of mortality at 1 year was increased by 123% when compared with those who were treated with oral agents.[82] A total

of 1181 patients with type 2 DM discharged after an MI were followed up for a median duration of 2.1 years in the DIGAMI (Diabetes Mellitus, Insulin Glucose Infusion in Acute Myocardial Infarction) 2 trial, of which 58% were on insulin. A post hoc proportional hazards regression analysis showed that although cardiovascular mortality was not affected, the risk of nonfatal MI and stroke was 73% higher in patients who were on insulin, and these differences persisted on separate analyses of patients for whom insulin was newly started and in those randomly assigned to insulin in the study.[83]

Clinical trials investigating the use of insulin infusions in patients with acute MI as well as critically ill patients in intensive care units have also led to controversy and uncertainty. The infusion of glucose-insulin-potassium (GIK) infusions in patients with acute MI was thought to optimize glucose influx into ischemic cardiomyocytes, promote glycolysis, reduce the increased concentration of free fatty acid caused by increased lipolysis, and optimize potassium handling in the ischemic cardiomyocyte. Although small studies performed in the era before the introduction of reperfusion therapies for treatment of acute MI suggested a mortality benefit of GIK infusion, larger studies in the context of contemporary management of acute MI have been discouraging. The largest of these trials in the modern era is the CREATE-ECLA (Clinical Trial of Reviparin and Metabolic Modulation in Acute Myocardial Infarction Treatment Evaluation–Estudios Cardiológicos Latinoamérica) trial, which studied 20,201 patients with ST-elevation myocardial infarction (STEMI) presenting within 12 hours of symptoms onset and randomized them to receive either high-dose GIK infusion with usual care or usual care alone. At 30 days postrandomization, no significant effects on mortality or adverse cardiovascular events were seen with the use of GIK, and the neutral effect was consistent across prespecified subgroup analyses that included patients with and without DM.[84] The neutral effect of high-dose GIK infusion in patients with acute STEMI was also seen in a combined analysis of data from the CREATE-ECLA and OASIS (Organization for the Assessment of Strategies for Ischemic Syndromes) 6 trials. However, in these trials, the incidence of hyperglycemia, hyperkalemia, and net fluid gain were significantly higher in those who received GIK infusion and may have been directly associated with a slight increase in mortality seen with the use of GIK infusion within the first 3 days after administration.[85] A subsequent reanalysis of the data from the CREATE-ECLA trial showed that if the GIK infusion had not induced hyperglycemia, insulin administration may have reduced the relative risk of mortality by 22%.[86]

Recently, 3 large randomized trials have been performed to study the effect of intensive glycemic control on cardiovascular outcomes and mortality in patients with type 2 DM. The ACCORD (Action to Control Cardiovascular Risk in Diabetes) trial studied 10,251 patients with type 2 DM who had known CAD or who were at high risk for CAD and randomized them to an intensive treatment approach (target HbA_{1c} level ≤6%) or to a standard approach (target HbA_{1c} level, 7%–7.9%). A rapid decline in HbA_{1c} levels was seen in both groups, more so in the intensive treatment group (median drop from 8.1% to 6.4% in 1 year), and this was caused by increased exposure to all classes of antidiabetic drugs, including insulin (11,902 person-years vs 7842 person-years in the standard therapy group). After a mean follow-up of 3.5 years, the incidence of the primary composite end point (cardiovascular death, nonfatal MI, nonfatal stroke) was not significantly affected, but the intensive therapy led to an increased risk of death (HR, 1.22, $P = .04$) when compared with standard therapy. A nonsignificant 10% reduction in nonfatal MI was observed at study termination ($P = .16$). The risks of hypoglycemia requiring treatment as well as of significant (>10 kg) weight gain were significantly increased in the intensive therapy group. No single drug or drug combination was associated with the excess mortality seen, but these results led to the premature termination of this study.[87] The ADVANCE (Action in Diabetes and Vascular Disease: Preterax and Diamicron Modified Release Controlled Evaluation) study randomized 11,140 patients with type 2 DM to intensive glucose control with a target HbA_{1c} level of 6.5% or less using a combination of modified-release gliclazide and other drugs or to standard glucose control. After a 5-year median follow-up, the achieved mean HbA_{1c} levels in the intensive and standard therapy groups were 6.5% and 7.3%, respectively. Intensive therapy modestly reduced the incidence of the primary composite end point comprising of micro- and macrovascular end points by 10% ($P = .01$). The risk of microvascular events was reduced by 14% ($P = .01$), attributed to a 21% decrease in the incidence of nephropathy ($P = .006$), while retinopathy was not significantly affected ($P = .5$). The incidence of macrovascular events and mortality was not significantly affected by the use of intensive therapy.[88] The VADT (Veterans Affairs Diabetes Trial) enrolled 1791 veterans with uncontrolled type 2 DM and randomized them to an intensive glycemic control strategy with a target absolute HbA_{1c} level reduction of 1.5% versus standard care. Forty percent of these patients had established CVD, 80% had hypertension, and 50% had hyperlipidemia. The primary outcome was time to first occurrence of a major cardiovascular event (MI, stroke, cardiovascular death, CHF, surgery for peripheral vascular disease, inoperable CAD, or amputation for ischemic gangrene). Achieved median HbA_{1c} levels after a median duration of 5.6 years in the intensive and standard glycemic control groups were 6.9% and 8.4%, respectively. No significant effect of intensive therapy was seen on either the primary composite outcome or any of the individual study end points.[89] The overall cardiovascular event rate was much less than the predicted event rate, affecting the statistical power of this study. These studies have revealed the perils of overzealous glycemic control and have also shown that although some populations, such as younger individuals, those without established CVD, and those with a shorter duration of type 2 DM and lower baseline HbA_{1c} levels, may benefit from aggressive glucose lowering, caution needs to be exercised to prevent severe hypoglycemia and sharp declines in HbA_{1c} levels.[90–92]

Acarbose

α-Glucosidase inhibitors such as acarbose may be useful as add-on therapy to reduce postprandial glucose levels in those patients with type 2 DM who may have contraindications to other medications. Data linking glycemic control with these agents on micro- and macrovascular clinical outcomes is scarce. The STOP-NIDDM (Study to Prevent Non-Insulin-Dependent Diabetes Mellitus) trial enrolled 1429 patients with impaired glucose tolerance (IGT) who were randomized to acarbose (n = 714) or to matching placebo (n = 715) and followed up for a mean duration of 3.3 years.[93] The trial was primarily designed to study the effect of acarbose on prevention of development of diabetes in patients with IGT and was not powered to detect changes in major cardiovascular events and the development of hypertension, which were recorded and reported as secondary end points. This trial had a large drop-out rate; 24% of enrolled patients discontinued study medication during the trial period, mainly citing gastrointestinal side effects. Although the event rate was rather low (the annual incidence of cardiovascular events in the placebo group was only 1.4%), the use of acarbose was reported to significantly reduce the risk of major cardiovascular events (HR, 0.51, $P = .03$) and MI (HR, 0.09, $P = .02$).[94] The incidence of developing DM, the primary study end point, was significantly reduced by the use of acarbose, yielding a HR of 0.64 and an absolute risk reduction of 8.7%. In addition, the relative risk of developing hypertension was also significantly reduced, with a HR of 0.66 (P = .006) and an absolute risk reduction of 5.3%. Acarbose also had significant salutary effects on body mass index (BMI), waist circumference, systolic and diastolic blood pressure, and triglyceride levels. No data on microvascular outcomes were published from this study. The overall data collectively suggest that in those who can tolerate acarbose, this drug may act in concert with other, more potent antidiabetic agents to improve the metabolic profile of these patients and possibly contribute in reducing adverse cardiovascular events. However, these results require validation in larger clinical trials adequately powered for micro- and macrovascular clinical outcomes in patients with an established diagnosis of type 2 DM.

Multifactorial Intervention Approaches

There is widespread consensus that the management of type 2 DM requires a comprehensive multifactorial strategy that includes the use of antiplatelet, antihypertensive, and antidyslipidemic agents along with antidiabetic medications and lifestyle modifications comprising of diet, weight reduction, and exercise. However, the efficacy of such a structured multifactorial approach on glycemic control as well as clinical outcomes was unknown. A retrospective case-control study in 113 type 2 diabetic patients with micro- or macroalbuminuria studied the efficacy of a proprietary multifactorial intervention program, which included dietary and lifestyle modifications as well as regulation of blood pressure, blood glucose levels, and serum lipid levels to specific targets, on CVD and CKD outcomes during a period of 5 years. The odds of all-cause mortality and first MI were significantly reduced in the intervention group (P<.05 compared with the control group).[95] In the larger Steno-2 study, 160 patients with type 2 DM and microalbuminuria were randomized to an intensive regimen or to conventional therapy (n = 80 in each group). The intensively treated group received target-driven therapy in the setting of behavior modification, with defined targets for HbA$_{1c}$ level (<6.5%), fasting total serum cholesterol level (<175 mg/dL), fasting triglyceride level (<150 mg/dL), and systolic (<130 mm Hg) and diastolic blood pressure (<80 mm Hg). In addition, they received low-dose aspirin and a multiple vitamin supplement. After a mean treatment period of 7.8 years, participants were subsequently followed up for

another 5.5 years on average. The study found that systolic blood pressure (P<.001) and albuminuria (P = .007) were significantly reduced in the intensive intervention group. Twenty patients in the intensive treatment group developed DKD (defined as overt proteinuria) compared with 37 in the conventional group (RR, 0.44, P = .004). Only 1 patient in the intensive treatment group had progression to end-stage renal disease as compared with 6 patients in the conventional group (P = .04).[96] After a mean duration of 7.8 years, time-to-first-event analysis showed that the adjusted HR for the composite CVD end point (CVD death, nonfatal MI, nonfatal stroke, revascularization procedures, amputation) in the intensive intervention group was 0.47 (95% CI, 0.22–0.74, P = .01), yielding an impressive 20% absolute risk reduction for the primary composite end point with the intensive intervention strategy. The Kaplan-Meier curves for cumulative cardiovascular events began to separate after about 2 years and continued to diverge thereafter until the end of the observation period.[97] The curve for microvascular outcomes began to separate after a mean of about 3.8 years of intensive treatment, and these differences were maintained until 13.3 years. Moreover, the survival curves for the incidence of the primary end point in the 2 groups showed a divergence as early as 24 months and continued to separate until the end of the study. Although the study was not designed to identify which elements of the intensive treatment contributed to the beneficial effect seen, the investigators determined that the use of statins and antihypertensive agents may have had the greatest effect, followed by antidiabetic agents and aspirin, using risk calculators based on epidemiologic data from the UKPDS.

Incretin-based Therapies: Glucagonlike Peptide 1 Receptor Agonists and Dipeptidyl Peptidase IV Inhibitors

It has long been known that orally administered glucose generates a more potent insulinotropic response than an intravenous glucose infusion, and this phenomenon, called the incretin effect, is significantly blunted in patients with type 2 DM.[98] The 2 important hormones (incretins) responsible for this effect are glucagon-like peptide (GLP) 1 and gastric inhibitory polypeptide, and studies have shown that disturbances in incretin pathways play a role in the progression of type 2 DM.[99] Reduction in GLP-1 secretion has been demonstrated in patients with type 2 DM, but the metabolic effects of GLP-1 on insulin and glucagon secretion, as well as on gastric emptying, are preserved. Two therapeutic approaches have therefore been developed to increase the levels of GLP-1 in patients with type 2 DM; one approach is the administration of exogenous analogs of GLP-1 that have a longer half-life and are resistant to the exopeptidase (dipeptidyl peptidase [DPP] IV) that cleaves endogenous GLP-1 and the other approach is the inhibition of the DPP-IV exopeptidase to increase the levels of endogenous GLP-1.

Exenatide is a GLP-1 receptor agonist that received FDA approval in 2005 for the treatment of type 2 DM and has been shown to significantly and durably reduce HbA_{1c} levels for as long as 3.5 years[100] and also cause significant weight reduction (mean reductions up to 5.3 kg in 3.5 years) and rates of hypoglycemia comparable to metformin.[101] In addition to enhancing glucose-dependent insulin secretion, exenatide restores the impaired first-phase insulin response, suppresses inappropriate postprandial glucagon secretion, and slows the accelerated rate of gastric emptying in patients with type 2 DM, thereby reducing the extent of postprandial hyperglycemia. Liraglutide, another partly DPP-resistant GLP-1 receptor agonist, has also been shown to significantly reduce HbA_{1c} levels and cause more modest levels of weight reduction. Sitagliptin is a DPP-IV inhibitor and was approved by the FDA in 2006 as an adjunctive therapy to lifestyle modification in patients with type 2 DM. Saxagliptin, another DPP-IV inhibitor, was approved by the FDA in July 2009 for treatment of type 2 DM either as monotherapy or in combination, whereas vildagliptin, approved for use in the European Union and Latin America, is not yet available in the United States. Small efficacy trials show that these agents significantly reduce HbA_{1c} levels by about 0.67% to 1.0% in 52 weeks and have an overall neutral effect on body weight. A cumulative meta-analysis of published clinical trials revealed that incretin-based therapies significantly reduced HbA_{1c} levels when compared with placebo and were noninferior to other antidiabetic agents.[102]

Animal studies have shown that GLP-1 improves myocardial insulin sensitivity and glucose uptake, improves myocardial contractility, and reduces heart rate and systemic vascular resistance. GLP-1 also plays a role in ischemic preconditioning of the myocardium, inhibits apoptotic pathways, and reduces ischemia-reperfusion injury.[103] Both exenatide and liraglutide have been shown to reduce infarct size in animal models of ischemia-reperfusion injury.[104,105] In addition, exenatide has also been shown to reduce circulating C-reactive protein (CRP) levels, with the greatest reductions (up to 50%) seen in those with higher baseline CRP levels.[106] Both exenatide and liraglutide have been shown in clinical trials to significantly reduce blood pressure (predominantly systolic blood pressure).[107,108] Exenatide also reduced total cholesterol, LDL cholesterol, and triglyceride levels and raised HDL cholesterol levels in patients followed up to 3.5 years, an effect likely related to weight reduction rather than a direct effect on lipid metabolism.[100]

However, to date, no clinical trials designed to study the effect of incretin-based therapies on adverse cardiovascular or kidney events have been published. Although the dose of exenatide does not need adjustment in the presence of CKD, clinical experience with this agent in patients with CKD stage 4 or postrenal transplantation is very limited. The dose of sitagliptin needs to be adjusted in the presence of CKD. Current guidelines[109] place the GLP-1 receptor agonist exenatide as a tier 2 treatment for the management of patients with type 2 DM. Randomized clinical trials are needed to determine whether the salutary glycemic and metabolic effects of incretin-based therapies actually translate in reduction of major cardiovascular or kidney outcomes.

THERAPEUTIC LIFESTYLE CHANGES

Although most health care providers recommend modest weight reduction, exercise, and dietary modification to overweight and obese patients with type 2 DM, there is insufficient data linking adherence to these recommendations to the prevention of micro- and macrovascular complications. However, several studies have shown that even modest weight loss and exercise can prevent the occurrence of type 2 DM in patients with IGT,[110] and epidemiologic studies have shown that obesity per se contributes to the overall disease burden of type 2 DM and its complications, including mortality.[111] Clinical guidelines issued by various medical societies[3,112] recommend that obese patients with type 2 DM (BMI >30 kg/m^2) be counseled about weight reduction, with an emphasis on individualization of treatment approaches and goals, but these derive largely from extrapolation of data from studies such as the Diabetes Prevention Program. This landmark study followed up 3234 patients with IGT who were either overweight or obese and demonstrated that lifestyle intervention that included modest weight reduction (5%–10% of body weight) along with up to 150 minutes of moderate exercise per week significantly reduced the incidence of overt type 2 DM,[113] and long-term follow-up for as long as 10 years after initiation of lifestyle modification therapies have shown that such effects on diabetes prevention can be sustained.[114] Weight reduction has been shown to reduce proteinuria in DKD and non-DKD.[115] Modest weight reduction resulting from a combination of caloric restriction and increased physical activity has been shown to be associated with lowering of blood pressure, improvement in lipid profiles, reduction in vascular stiffness, as well as reduction in the circulating levels of inflammatory markers and measures of insulin resistance.[116–119] However, its effect on cardiac structure and function, as well as on the incidence of clinical events has not been conclusively shown, largely because of the short duration of follow-up in these and other studies.

From a practical standpoint, health care providers should continue to encourage their obese patients with type 2 DM to modify their diet, as well as engage in regular moderate aerobic or resistance exercise, with individualization of these approaches based on the patient's physical condition, values, and expectations. Overweight patients should be advised to avoid further weight gain so as to reduce the effects of adiposity on various metabolic parameters, such as inflammation, insulin resistance, lipid metabolism, and blood pressure. A reasonable approach would be to advise patients to reduce their caloric intake by about 500 kcal a day, with the aim of losing approximately 1 lb (450 g) per week. Because the effect on glycemic control is primarily determined by total carbohydrate intake, up to 60% of nonprotein calories should be derived from complex carbohydrates.[120] In addition, adequate dietary fiber intake should also be encouraged, along with an emphasis on meeting the recommended daily allowance of fruits and vegetables. More research is needed to determine the effect of these approaches on hard clinical outcomes of micro- and macrovascular disease in patients with type 2 DM.

EMERGING DRUG CLASSES FOR THE TREATMENT OF DIABETIC VASCULAR COMPLICATIONS AND HYPERGLYCEMIA
Protein kinase C Inhibitors

The protein kinase C (PKC) family has been identified as an important mediator of hyperglycemia-induced cellular damage and is implicated in the pathogenesis of diabetic complications. This group of kinases consists of at least 10 distinct isoforms, but animal studies have shown that PKCα and PKCβ are the major isoforms involved in the causation of diabetic complications. In the kidney, PKCα seems to be important in regulation of the glomerular barrier and thereby UAE, whereas PKCβ is involved in the development of renal and glomerular hypertrophy as well as mesangial expansion.[121] PKCα is the predominant isoform in the heart of a diabetic adult and is implicated in the maladaptive cardiac remodeling seen in diabetic heart failure; overexpression of PKCα has been shown to blunt myocardial contractility in a murine model of heart failure.[122] More recent research has also shown that inhibition of PKC using ruboxistaurin attenuated cardiomyocyte hypertrophy and collagen deposition and preserved diastolic function and cardiac contractility in a rodent model of diabetic heart failure.[123] Ruboxistaurin is a selective PKCβ inhibitor and has been studied in patients with microvascular diabetic complications such as nephropathy and retinopathy. A pilot, phase 2, placebo-controlled trial in patients with type 2 DM and macroalbuminuria showed that ruboxistaurin reduced albuminuria, rate of eGFR decline, and urinary transforming growth factor (TGF) β excretion.[124,125] A larger post hoc analysis of 1157 patients with diabetic retinopathy who were either randomized to ruboxistaurin or to placebo and followed up for an average of at least 3 years showed that selective PKCβ inhibition with ruboxistaurin did not have an adverse safety profile, but the available data were insufficient to determine benefits of ruboxistaurin on albuminuria, eGFR, or clinical end points.[126] As such, additional clinical trial evidence for safety and efficacy are necessary before this agent can be indicated for DKD. Current research is also focusing on the development of different agents with selectivities for other PKC isoforms, including PKCα, as well as formulation of novel drug delivery systems for organ-specific delivery of these agents.[127]

Advanced Glycation End Product Inhibitors

Advanced glycation end products (AGEs) are a heterogeneous group of compounds that are formed by the nonenzymatic reaction between reducing sugars and amine residues on proteins, nucleic acids, and lipids. They may originate from exogenous sources such as AGE-rich foods and tobacco smoke or may be endogenously produced by the body. These substances accumulate in various tissues, and this accumulation is increased in diabetic patients because of increased AGE formation attributable to chronic hyperglycemia and activation of inflammatory mediators and reactive oxygen species, as well as reduced enzymatic degradation and reduced renal clearance of these compounds. A large body of evidence has linked AGEs to the pathogenesis of cardiovascular and kidney disease in diabetes. AGEs exert their deleterious effects by induction of cross-linking of structural proteins, such as collagen and other extracellular matrix proteins, as well as stimulation of a host of secondary messenger pathways leading to activation of protein kinases and generation of reactive oxygen species, proinflammatory cytokines, and growth factors by interaction with specialized receptors for AGEs and other receptors.[128] Various therapeutic agents have been developed that are inhibitors of AGE formation (aminoguanidine, pyridoxamine, OPB-9195, LR-90, PARP inhibitors), breakers of cross-links (ALT-711/alagebrium), and inhibitors of dietary AGE absorption (AST-120). Most of these agents have been studied in vitro or in animal models of DM. Aminoguanidine entered clinical trials in the early 1990s, but drug development was halted because of safety concerns (CVD and systemic vasculitis) and inconclusive data for efficacy in DKD.[129,130] Pyridoxamine continues to be studied actively in clinical studies, and early phase 2 evaluations in diabetic patients with overt nephropathy have shown that the rate of increase in serum creatinine levels and urinary excretion of TGF-β were blunted after 24 weeks of pyridoxamine therapy.[131] As is the case with ruboxistaurin, further study with large-scale, prospective clinical trials are needed to confirm the safety and efficacy of pyridoxamine.

Sodium-Glucose Cotransporter 2 Inhibitors

Sodium-glucose cotransporters (SGLTs) are a group of transporter proteins that cotransport glucose and sodium intracellularly using the sodium-potassium gradient generated by the sodium-potassium adenosine triphosphatase pumps in the basolateral membrane of the cell. The SGLT2 isoform is expressed in the S1 and S2 segments of the proximal convoluted tubules and is responsible for about 90% of reabsorption of glucose in the kidney.[132,133] In patients with uncontrolled diabetes, there is upregulation of SGLT2 expression in the kidney to preserve the glucose reabsorptive capacity of the kidney in the setting of hyperglycemia.[134,135] However, observations in persons with inherited mutations of the SLC5A2 gene, which encodes the SGLT2 receptor, as well as early experiments with phlorizin (a competitive inhibitor of sodium-glucose cotransport in renal and epithelial cells) have shown that SGLT inhibition can lower ambient blood glucose levels and improve counter-regulatory responses without affecting insulin levels.[136] Selective SGLT2 inhibitors currently in development are O-glucosides (remogliflozin etabonate, sergliflozin) or C-aryl glucosides (dapagliflozin), which are competitive inhibitors of the SGLT2 receptor, and, more recently, antisense oligonucleotides such as ISIS 388626 and ISIS-SGLT2$_{RX}$, which reduce the expression of the SGLT2 gene. Remogliflozin etabonate and AVE2268 are at present being studied in phase 2 clinical trials. Dapagliflozin has been shown to cause significant dose-dependent reductions in FPG levels and concomitant increase in glucosuria in phase 2 clinical studies, and 2 larger, phase 3 randomized clinical trials (registered on http://www.clinicaltrials.gov as NCT00528372 and NCT00528879) are currently underway to study its efficacy in drug-naive and metformin-treated patients with type 2 DM.[137] Concerns with the use of these drugs include their long-term effects on fluid and electrolyte balance, bone health, and a possible increase in the incidence of urinary tract infections and genital fungal infections. In addition to the study of these agents expressly for treatment of hyperglycemia, it will be important to assess effects on relevant clinical end points related to CVD and DKD.

SUMMARY

The prevalence of DM and its vascular complications continues to increase worldwide. A wide array of therapeutic agents are now available for the treatment of hyperglycemia, and large randomized clinical trials using these agents have provided valuable insight not only into their effects on glycemic control and on the risk of diabetic complications but also into the disease process itself. Results of recently completed clinical trials have shed new light on the perils of aggressive glycemic control in patients with type 2 DM with currently available agents and have confirmed previously observed differences in the effects of glycemic control on micro-and macrovascular complications. A multifactorial approach to the treatment of DM should incorporate the use of antihyperglycemic agents, alone or in combination, for steady and sustained glycemic control, along with lifestyle modification including dietary adjustment and regular exercise, as well as treatment of concomitant hypertension and hyperlipidemia. New drug classes are being developed to target novel molecular pathways for the treatment of hyperglycemia as well as for the prevention of diabetic vascular complications, and studies using many of these agents are ongoing.

REFERENCES

1. World Health Organization. Fact sheet no. 312: what is diabetes? Available at: http://www.who.int/mediacentre/factsheets/fs312/en/. Accessed October 16, 2009.

2. Wild S, Roglic G, Green A, et al. Global prevalence of diabetes: estimates for the year 2000 and projections for 2030. Diabetes Care 2004;27(5): 1047–53.

3. National Kidney Foundation – Kidney Disease Outcomes Quality Initiative (NKF-KDOQI). Clinical practice guidelines and clinical practice recommendations for diabetes and chronic kidney disease. Am J Kidney Dis 2007;49:S1–179.

4. American Heart Association. Heart disease and stroke statistics-2008 update: a report from the American Heart Association Statistics Committee and Stroke Statistics Subcommittee. Circulation 2008;117(4):e25–146.

5. Nathan DM, Zinman B, Cleary PA, et al. Diabetes Control and Complications Trial/Epidemiology of Diabetes Interventions and Complications (DCCT/EDIC) Research Group. Modern-day clinical course of type 1 diabetes mellitus after 30 years' duration: the diabetes control and complications trial/epidemiology of diabetes interventions and complications and Pittsburgh epidemiology of diabetes complications experience (1983–2005). Arch Intern Med 2009;169(14):1307–16.

6. Holman RR, Paul SK, Bethel MA, et al. 10-year follow-up of intensive glucose control in type 2 diabetes. N Engl J Med 2008;359(15):1577–89.

7. U.S. Renal Data System, USRDS 2009. Annual data report: Atlas of chronic kidney disease and end-stage renal disease in the United States. Bethesda (MD): National Institutes of Health, National Institute of Diabetes and Digestive and Kidney Diseases. 2009. Available at: http://www.usrds.org/2009/view/v1_00a_intro.asp. Accessed January 11, 2010.

8. Adler A, Stevens R, Manley S, et al. Development and progression of nephropathy in type 2 diabetes: The United Kingdom Prospective Diabetes Study (UKPDS 64). Kidney Int 2003;63: 225–32.

9. International Diabetes Federation. The human, social and economic impact of diabetes. Available at: http://www.idf.org/home/index.cfm?node=41./. Accessed October 16, 2009.

10. Wiernsperger NF, Bailey CJ. The antihyperglycaemic effect of metformin: therapeutic and cellular mechanisms. Drugs 1999;58(Suppl 1):31–9.

11. University Group Diabetes Program. A study of the effects of hypoglycemic agents on vascular complications on patients with adult-onset diabetes: V. evaluation of phenformin therapy. Diabetes 1975;24(Suppl 1):65–184.

12. Stang M, Wysowski DK, Butler-Jones D. Incidence of lactic acidosis in metformin users. Diabetes Care 1999;22:925–7.

13. Davidson MB, Peters AL. An overview of metformin in the treatment of type 2 diabetes mellitus. Am J Med 1997;102:99–110.

14. DeFronzo R. Pharmacologic therapy for type 2 diabetes mellitus. Ann Intern Med 1999;131: 281–303.

15. National Kidney Foundation. KDOQI clinical practice guidelines for chronic kidney disease: evaluation, classification, and stratification. Available at: http://www.kidney.org/Professionals/Kdoqi/guidelines_ckd/toc.htm. Accessed January 11, 2010.

16. Effect of intensive blood-glucose control with metformin on complications in overweight patients with type 2 diabetes (UKPDS 34). UK Prospective Diabetes Study (UKPDS) Group. Lancet 1998; 352:854–65 [erratum in: Lancet 1998;352:1558].

17. Inzucchi SE. Metformin for heart failure-innocent until proven guilty. Diabetes Care 2005;28: 2585–7.

18. Misbin RI, Green L, Stadel BV, et al. Lactic acidosis in patients with diabetes treated with metformin. N Engl J Med 1998;338:265–6.

19. Rachmani R, Slavachevski I, Levi Z, et al. Metformin in patients with type 2 diabetes mellitus: reconsideration of traditional contraindications. Eur J Intern Med 2002;13:428–33.

20. Eurich DT, Majumdar SR, McAlister FA, et al. Improved clinical outcomes associated with metformin in patients with diabetes and heart failure. Diabetes Care 2005;28:2345–51.

21. Inzucchi SE, Masoudi FA, Wang Y, et al. Insulin-sensitizing antihyperglycemic drugs and mortality after acute myocardial infarction: insights from the National Heart Care Project. Diabetes Care 2005; 28:1680–9.

22. Cryer DR, Nicholas SP, Henry DH, et al. Comparative outcomes study of metformin intervention versus conventional approach-the COSMIC Approach Study. Diabetes Care 2005;28:539–43.

23. Eurich DT. Metformin treatment in diabetes and heart failure: when academic equipoise meets clinical reality. Trials 2009;10:12.

24. Masoudi FA, Wang Y, Inzucchi SE, et al. Metformin and thiazolidinedione use in Medicare patients with heart failure. JAMA 2003;290:81–5.

25. MicroMedex. DrugPoint Summary-Metformin hydrochloride-dosing and indications. Available at: http://www.micromedex.com/products/drugdex/. Accessed November 9, 2009.

26. Meinert CL, Knatterud GL, Prout TE, et al. A study of the effects of hypoglycemic agents on vascular complications in patients with adult-onset diabetes. II. Mortality results. Diabetes 1970;19(Suppl):789–830.

27. Murry CE, Jennings RB, Reimer KA. Preconditioning with ischemia: a delay in lethal injury in ischemic myocardium. Circulation 1986;24:1124–6.

28. Chutkow WA, Simon MC, Le Beau MM, et al. Cloning, tissue expression, and chromosomal localization of SUR2, the putative drug-binding

subunit of cardiac, skeletal muscle, and vascular KATP channels. Diabetes 1996;45:1439–45.

29. Lawrence CL, Proks P, Rodrigo GC, et al. Gliclazide produces a high-affinity block of KATP channels in mouse isolated pancreatic beta cells but not rat heart or arterial smooth muscle cells. Diabetologia 2001;44:1019–25.

30. Legtenberg RJ, Houston RJ, Oeseburg B, et al. Effects of sulfonylurea derivatives on ischemia-induced loss of function in the isolated rat heart. Eur J Pharmacol 2001;419:85–92.

31. Dobrowski M, Wahl P, Holmes WE, et al. Effect of repaglinide on cloned beta cell, cardiac and smooth muscle types of ATP-sensitive potassium channels. Diabetologia 2001;44:747–56.

32. Lee TM, Chou TF. Impairment of myocardial protection in type 2 diabetic patients. J Clin Endocrinol Metab 2003;88:531–7.

33. Intensive blood-glucose control with sulphonylureas or insulin compared with conventional treatment and risk of complications in patients with type 2 diabetes (UKPDS 33). UK Prospective Diabetes Study (UKPDS) Group. Lancet 1998;352:837–53 [erratum in: Lancet 1999;354: 602].

34. Kahn SE, Haffner SM, Heise MA, et al. ADOPT Study Group. Glycemic durability of rosiglitazone, metformin, or glyburide monotherapy. N Engl J Med 2006;355:2427–43 [erratum in: N Engl J Med 2007;356:1387–8].

35. Simpson S, Majumdar S, Tsuyuki RT, et al. Dose-response relation between sulphonylurea drugs and mortality in type 2 diabetes mellitus: a population-based cohort study. CMAJ 2006;174(2):169–74.

36. Black C, Donnelly P, McIntyre L, et al. Meglitinide analogues for type 2 diabetes mellitus. Cochrane Database Syst Rev 2007;2:CD00004654.

37. Johansen OE, Birkeland KI. Defining the role of repaglinide in the management of type 2 diabetes mellitus-a review. Am J Cardiovasc Drugs 2007; 7(5):319–35.

38. Hasslacher C. Safety and efficacy of repaglinide in type 2 diabetic patients with and without impaired renal function. Diabetes Care 2003;26:886–91.

39. Schumacher S, Abbasi I, Weise D, et al. Single- and multiple-dose pharmacokinetics of repaglinide in patients with type 2 diabetes and renal impairment. Eur J Clin Pharmacol 2001;57:147–52.

40. Willson TM, Brown PJ, Sternbach DD, et al. The PPARs: from orphan receptors to drug discovery. J Med Chem 2000;43:527–50.

41. Spiegelman BM. PPAR-gamma: adipogenic regulator and thiazolidinedione receptor. Diabetes 1998;47:507–14.

42. Sarafidis PA, Bakris GL. Protection of the kidney by thiazolidinediones: an assessment from bench to bedside. Kidney Int 2006;70:1223–33.

43. Dormandy JA, Charbonnel B, Eckland DJ, et al. PROactive investigators. Secondary prevention of macrovascular events in patients with type 2 diabetes in the PROactive Study (PROspective pioglitAzone Clinical Trial In macroVascular Events): a randomised controlled trial. Lancet 2005; 366(9493):1279–89.

44. Lebovitz HE, Dole JF, Patwardhan R, et al. Rosiglitazone monotherapy is effective in patients with type 2 diabetes. J Clin Endocrinol Metab 2001;86:280–8.

45. Bakris G, Viberti G, Weston WM, et al. Rosiglitazone reduces urinary albumin excretion in type 2 diabetes. J Hum Hypertens 2003;17:7–12.

46. Aljabri K, Kozak SE, Thompson DM. Addition of pioglitazone or bedtime insulin to maximal doses of sulfonylurea and metformin in type 2 diabetes patients with poor glucose control: a prospective, randomized trial. Am J Med 2004;116:230–5.

47. Hanefeld M, Brunetti P, Schernthaner GH, et al. One-year glycemic control with a sulfonylurea plus pioglitazone versus a sulfonylurea plus metformin in patients with type 2 diabetes. Diabetes Care 2004;27:141–7.

48. Schernthaner G, Matthews DR, Charbonnel B, et al. Efficacy and safety of pioglitazone versus metformin in patients with type 2 diabetes mellitus: a double-blind, randomized trial. J Clin Endocrinol Metab 2004;89:6068–76.

49. Matthews DR, Charbonnel BH, Hanefeld M, et al. Long-term therapy with addition of pioglitazone to metformin compared with the addition of gliclazide to metformin in patients with type 2 diabetes: a randomized, comparative study. Diabetes Metab Res Rev 2005;21:167–74.

50. Bakris GL, Ruilope LM, McMorn SO, et al. Rosiglitazone reduces microalbuminuria and blood pressure independently of glycemia in type 2 diabetes patients with microalbuminuria. J Hypertens 2006;24:2047–55.

51. Ryan EH Jr, Han DP, Ramsay RC, et al. Diabetic macular edema associated with glitazone use. Retina 2006;26:562–70.

52. ACTOS (pioglitazone hydrochloride) - full prescribing information and medication guide. Available at: http://www.actos.com/actospro/prescribinginfo.aspx. Accessed January 11, 2010.

53. Avandia (rosiglitazone maleate) prescribing information. Available at: http://us.gsk.com/products/assets/us_avandia.pdf. Accessed January 11, 2010.

54. Koshiyama H, Shimono D, Kuwamura N, et al. Rapid communication: inhibitory effect of pioglitazone on carotid arterial wall thickness in type 2 diabetes. J Clin Endocrinol Metab 2001;86:3452–6.

55. Langenfeld MR, Forst T, Hohberg C, et al. Pioglitazone decreases carotid intima-media thickness independently of glycemic control in patients with

type 2 diabetes mellitus: results from a controlled randomized study. Circulation 2005;111:2525–31.

56. Mazzone T, Meyer PM, Feinstein SB, et al. Effect of pioglitazone compared with glimepiride on carotid intima-media thickness in type 2 diabetes: a randomized trial. JAMA 2006;296:2572–81.

57. Takagi T, Yamamuro A, Tamita K, et al. Pioglitazone reduces neointimal tissue proliferation after coronary stent implantation in patients with type 2 diabetes mellitus: an intravascular ultrasound scanning study. Am Heart J 2003;146:e5.

58. Riche DM, Valderrama R, Henyan NN. Thiazolidinediones and risk of repeat target vessel revascularization following percutaneous coronary intervention: a meta-analysis. Diabetes Care 2007;30(2):384–8.

59. Gerstein HC, Yusuf S, Bosch J, et al. DREAM (Diabetes REduction Assessment with Ramipril and Rosiglitazone Medication) Trial Investigators. Effect of rosiglitazone on the frequency of diabetes in patients with impaired glucose tolerance or impaired fasting glucose: a randomized controlled trial. Lancet 2006;368:1096–105.

60. Nissen SE, Wolski K. Effect of rosiglitazone on the risk of myocardial infarction and death from cardiovascular causes. N Engl J Med 2007;356:2457–71.

61. Lipscombe LL, Gomes T, Lévesque LE, et al. Thiazolidinediones and cardiovascular outcomes in older patients with diabetes. JAMA 2007;298: 2634–43.

62. Singh S, Loke YK, Furberg CD. Long-term risk of cardiovascular events with rosiglitazone: a meta-analysis. JAMA 2007;298:1189–95.

63. Richter B, Bandeira-Echtler E, Bergerhoff K, et al. Rosiglitazone for type 2 diabetes mellitus. Cochrane Database Syst Rev 2007;3:CD006063.

64. Mannucci E, Monami M, Di Bari M, et al. Cardiac safety profile of rosiglitazone. A comprehensive meta-analysis of randomized clinical trials. Int J Cardiol 2009. [Epub ahead of print].

65. Friedrich JO, Beyene J, Adhikari NK. Rosiglitazone: can meta-analysis accurately estimate excess cardiovascular risk given the available data? Re-analysis of randomized trials using various methodologic approaches. BMC Res Notes 2009;2:5.

66. Lincoff AM, Wolski K, Nicholls SJ, et al. Pioglitazone and risk of cardiovascular events in patients with type 2 diabetes mellitus: a meta-analysis of randomized trials. JAMA 2007;298(10):1180–8.

67. Mannucci E, Monami M, Lamanna C, et al. Pioglitazone and cardiovascular risk-a comprehensive meta-analysis of randomized clinical trials. Diabetes Obes Metab 2008;10:1221–38.

68. Nagajothi N, Adigopula S, Balamuthusamy S, et al. Pioglitazone and the risk of myocardial infarction and other major adverse cardiac events: a meta-analysis of randomized, controlled trials. Am J Ther 2008;15:506–11.

69. Diamond GA, Bax L, Kaul S. Uncertain effects of rosiglitazone on the risk for myocardial infarction and cardiovascular death. Ann Intern Med 2007; 147:578–81.

70. Fuster V, Farkouh ME. Faster publication isn't always better. Nat Clin Pract Cardiovasc Med 2007;4:345.

71. Mulrow CD, Cornell J, Localio AR. Rosiglitazone: a thunderstorm from scarce and fragile data. Ann Intern Med 2007;147:585–7.

72. A desktop guide to type 2 diabetes mellitus: European Diabetes Policy Group 1999. Diabet Med 1999;16:716–30.

73. Erdmann E, Dormandy JA, Charbonnel B, et al. PROactive Investigators. The effect of pioglitazone on recurrent myocardial infarction in 2,445 patients with type 2 diabetes and previous myocardial infarction: results from the PROactive (PROactive 05) Study. J Am Coll Cardiol 2007;49:1772–80.

74. Pioglitazone protects DM patients against re-infarction (PPAR Study). (NCT00212004). Available at: http://www.clinicaltrials.gov/ct2/show/NCT00212004?term=NCT00212004&rank=1. Accessed January 11, 2010.

75. Cobitz A, Zambanini A, Sowell M, et al. A retrospective evaluation of congestive heart failure and myocardial ischemia events in 14,237 patients with type 2 diabetes mellitus enrolled in 42 short-term, double-blind, randomized clinical studies with rosiglitazone. Pharmacoepidemiol Drug Saf 2008;17:769–81.

76. Walker AM, Koro CE, Landon J. Coronary heart disease outcomes in patients receiving antidiabetic agents in the PharMetrics database 2000–2007. Pharmacoepidemiol Drug Saf 2008;17(8): 760–8.

77. Home PD, Pocock SJ, Beck-Nielsen H, et al. RECORD Study Team. Rosiglitazone evaluated for cardiovascular outcomes in oral agent combination therapy for type 2 diabetes (RECORD): a multicentre, randomised, open-label trial. Lancet 2009; 373:2125–35.

78. The effect of intensive treatment of diabetes on the development and progression of long-term complications in insulin-dependent diabetes mellitus. The Diabetes Control and Complications Trial Research Group. N Engl J Med 1993;329:977–86.

79. Nathan DM, Cleary PA, Backlund JY, et al. Diabetes Control and Complications Trial/Epidemiology of Diabetes Interventions and Complications (DCCT/EDIC) Study Research Group. Intensive diabetes treatment and cardiovascular disease in patients with type 1 diabetes. N Engl J Med 2005;353: 2643–53.

80. Khaw KT, Wareham N, Bingham S, et al. Association of hemoglobin A1c with cardiovascular disease and mortality in adults: the European

prospective investigation into cancer in Norfolk. Ann Intern Med 2004;141:413–20.

81. Dandona P, Chaudhuri A, Ghanim H, et al. Use of insulin to improve glycemic control in diabetes mellitus. Cardiovasc Drugs Ther 2008;22:241–51.

82. Anselmino M, Ohrvik J, Malmberg K, et al. Euro Heart Survey Investigators. Glucose lowering treatment in patients with coronary artery disease is prognostically important not only in established but also in newly detected diabetes mellitus: a report from the Euro Heart Survey on Diabetes and the Heart. Eur Heart J 2008;29:177–84.

83. Mellbin LG, Malmberg K, Norhammar A, et al. DIGAMI 2 Investigators. The impact of glucose lowering treatment on long-term prognosis in patients with type 2 diabetes and myocardial infarction: a report from the DIGAMI 2 trial. Eur Heart J 2008;29:166–76.

84. Mehta SR, Yusuf S, Díaz R, et al. CREATE-ECLA Trial Group Investigators. Effect of glucose-insulin-potassium infusion on mortality in patients with acute ST-segment elevation myocardial infarction: the CREATE-ECLA randomized controlled trial. JAMA 2005;293(4):437–46.

85. Díaz R, Goyal A, Mehta SR, et al. Glucose-insulin-potassium therapy in patients with ST-segment elevation myocardial infarction. JAMA 2007; 298(20):2399–405.

86. Chaudhuri A, Miller M, Nesto R, et al. Targeting glucose in acute myocardial infarction: has glucose, insulin, and potassium infusion missed the target. Diabetes Care 2007;30:3026–8.

87. Gerstein HC, Miller ME, Byington RP, et al. Action to Control Cardiovascular Risk in Diabetes Study Group. Effects of intensive glucose lowering in type 2 diabetes. N Engl J Med 2008;358:2545–59.

88. Patel A, MacMahon S, Chalmers J, et al. ADVANCE Collaborative Group. Intensive blood glucose control and vascular outcomes in patients with type 2 diabetes. N Engl J Med 2008;358:2560–72.

89. Duckworth W, Abraira C, Moritz T, et al. VADT Investigators. Glucose control and vascular complications in veterans with type 2 diabetes. N Engl J Med 2009;360:129–39.

90. Skyler JS, Bergenstal R, Bonow RO, et al. Intensive glycemic control and the prevention of cardiovascular events: implications of the ACCORD, ADVANCE, and VA Diabetes Trials: a position statement of the American Diabetes Association and a Scientific Statement of the American College of Cardiology Foundation and the American Heart Association. J Am Coll Cardiol 2009;53:298–304.

91. Dluhy RG, McMahon GT. Intensive glycemic control in the ACCORD and ADVANCE trials. N Engl J Med 2008;358:2630–3.

92. Cefalu WT. Glycemic targets and cardiovascular disease. N Engl J Med 2008;358:2633–5.

93. Chiasson JL, Josse RG, Gomis R, et al. STOP-NIDDM Trial Research Group. Acarbose treatment and the risk of cardiovascular disease and hypertension in patients with impaired glucose tolerance: the STOP-NIDDM trial. JAMA 2003;290:486–94.

94. Chiasson JL. Acarbose for the prevention of diabetes, hypertension, and cardiovascular disease in subjects with impaired glucose tolerance: the Study to Prevent Non-Insulin-Dependent Diabetes Mellitus (STOP-NIDDM) Trial. Endocr Pract 2006; 12(Suppl 1):25–30.

95. Steines W, Piehlmeier W, Schenkirsch G, et al. Effectiveness of a disease management programme for patients with type 2 diabetes mellitus and albuminuria in primary care - the PROSIT project (Proteinuria Screening and Intervention). Exp Clin Endocrinol Diabetes 2004;112:88–94.

96. Gaede P, Lund-Anderson H, Parving HH, et al. Effect of a multifactorial intervention on mortality in type 2 diabetes. N Engl J Med 2008;358:580–91.

97. Gaede P, Vedel P, Larsen N, et al. Multifactorial intervention and cardiovascular disease in patients with type 2 diabetes. N Engl J Med 2003;348: 383–93.

98. Nauck M, Stöckmann F, Ebert R, et al. Reduced incretin effect in type 2 (non-insulin-dependent) diabetes. Diabetologia 1986;29:46–52.

99. Drucker DJ, Nauck MA. The incretin system: glucagon-like peptide-1 receptor agonists and dipeptidyl peptidase-4 inhibitors in type 2 diabetes. Lancet 2006;368:1696–705.

100. Klonoff DC, Buse JB, Nielsen LL, et al. Exenatide effects on diabetes, obesity, cardiovascular risk factors and hepatic biomarkers in patients with type 2 diabetes treated for at least 3 years. Curr Med Res Opin 2008;24:275–86.

101. Bolen S, Feldman L, Vassy J, et al. Systematic review: comparative effectiveness and safety of oral medications for type 2 diabetes mellitus. Ann Intern Med 2007;147:386–99.

102. Amori RE, Lau J, Pittas AG. Efficacy and safety of incretin therapy in type 2 diabetes: systematic review and meta-analysis. JAMA 2007;298: 194–206.

103. Sulistio M, Carothers C, Mangat M, et al. GLP-1 agonist-based therapies: an emerging new class of antidiabetic drug with potential cardioprotective effects. Curr Atheroscler Rep 2009;11:93–9.

104. Sonne DP, Engstrom T, Treiman M. Protective effects of GLP-1 analogues exendin-4 and GLP-1(9-36) amide against ischemia-reperfusion injury in rat heart. Regul Pept 2008;146:243–9.

105. Noyan-Ashraf MH, Ban K, Sadi A, et al. The GLP-1R agonist liraglutide protects cardiomyocytes and improves survival and cardiac function after experimental murine infarction [abstract 190-OR]. Presented at the 68th scientific sessions of the

American Diabetes Association. San Francisco (CA), June 6–10, 2008.

106. Kendall DM, Bhole D, Guan X, et al. Exenatide treatment for 82 weeks reduced C-reactive protein, HbA1c, and body weight in patients with type 2 diabetes mellitus. Presented at 42nd Congress of EASD. Copenhagen (Denmark), September 14–17, 2006.

107. Okerson T, Yan P, Stonehouse A, et al. Exenatide improved systolic blood pressure compared to insulin or placebo in patients with type 2 diabetes [abstract 877]. Presented at the 44th Annual meeting of the EASD. Rome (Italy), September 7–11, 2008.

108. Colagiuri S, Frid A, Zdravkovic M, et al. Liraglutide, a human GLP-1 analogue, reduces systolic blood pressure in subjects with type 2 diabetes in subjects with type 2 diabetes [abstract 899]. Presented at the 44th Annual meeting of the EASD. Rome (Italy), September 7–11, 2008.

109. Nathan DM, Buse JB, Davidson MB, et al. Medical management of hyperglycemia in type 2 diabetes: a consensus algorithm for the initiation and adjustment of therapy: a consensus statement of the American Diabetes Association and the European Association for the Study of Diabetes. Diabetes Care 2009;32:193–203.

110. Roumen C, Blaak EE, Corpeleijn E. Lifestyle intervention for prevention of diabetes: determinants of success for future implementation. Nutr Rev 2009;67:132–46.

111. Flegal KM, Graubard BI, Williamson DF, et al. Cause-specific excess deaths associated with underweight, overweight, and obesity. JAMA 2007;298:2028–37.

112. Snow V, Barry P, Fitterman N, et al. Clinical Efficacy Assessment Subcommittee of the American College of Physicians. Pharmacologic and surgical management of obesity in primary care: a clinical practice guideline from the American College of Physicians. Ann Intern Med 2005;142:525–31.

113. Knowler WC, Barrett-Connor E, Fowler SE, et al. Diabetes Prevention Program Research Group. Reduction in the incidence of type 2 diabetes with lifestyle intervention or metformin. N Engl J Med 2002;346:393–403.

114. Diabetes Prevention Program Research Group. 10-year follow-up of diabetes incidence and weight loss in the Diabetes Prevention Program Outcomes Study. Lancet 2009;374:1677–86.

115. Morales E, Valero MA, Leon M, et al. Beneficial effects of weight loss in overweight patients with chronic proteinuric nephropathies. Am J Kidney Dis 2003;41:319–27.

116. Reid CM, Dart AM, Dewar EM, et al. Interactions between the effects of exercise and weight loss on risk factors, cardiovascular haemodynamics and left ventricular structure in overweight subjects. J Hypertens 1994;12(3):291–301.

117. Esposito K, Pontillo A, Di Palo C, et al. Effect of weight loss and lifestyle changes on vascular inflammatory markers in obese women: a randomized trial. JAMA 2003;289(14):1799–804.

118. Skilton MR, Sieveking DP, Harmer JA, et al. The effects of obesity and non-pharmacological weight loss on vascular and ventricular function and structure. Diabetes Obes Metab 2008;10(10):874–84.

119. Goldberg Y, Boaz M, Matas Z, et al. Weight loss induced by nutritional and exercise intervention decreases arterial stiffness in obese subjects. Clin Nutr 2009;28(1):21–5.

120. National Academy of Sciences, Institute of Medicine. Dietary reference intakes for energy, carbohydrates, fiber, fat, fatty acids, cholesterol, protein and amino acids (Macronutrients). Washington, DC: The National Academy Press; 2002. Chapter 8.

121. Menne J, Meier M, Park JK, et al. Inhibition of protein kinase C in diabetic nephropathy–where do we stand? Nephrol Dial Transplant 2009;24:2021–3.

122. Hambleton M, Hahn H, Pleger ST, et al. Pharmacological- and gene therapy-based inhibition of protein kinase C alpha/beta enhances cardiac contractility and attenuates heart failure. Circulation 2006;114:574–82.

123. Connelly KA, Kelly DJ, Zhang Y, et al. Inhibition of protein kinase C-beta by ruboxistaurin preserves cardiac function and reduces extracellular matrix production in diabetic cardiomyopathy. Circ Heart Fail 2009;2:129–37.

124. Tuttle KR, Bakris GL, Toto RD, et al. The effect of ruboxistaurin on nephropathy in type 2 diabetes. Diabetes Care 2005;28:2686–90.

125. Gilbert RE, Kim SA, Tuttle KR, et al. Effect of ruboxistaurin on urinary transforming growth factor-beta in patients with diabetic nephropathy and type 2 diabetes. Diabetes Care 2007;30:995–6.

126. Tuttle KR, McGill JB, Haney DJ, et al. Kidney outcomes in long-term studies of ruboxistaurin for diabetic eye disease. Clin J Am Soc Nephrol 2007;2:631–6.

127. Palaniyandi SS, Sun L, Ferreira JC, et al. Protein kinase C in heart failure: a therapeutic target? Cardiovasc Res 2009;82:229–39.

128. Goh SY, Cooper ME. Clinical review: the role of advanced glycation end products in progression and complications of diabetes. J Clin Endocrinol Metab 2008;93:1143–52.

129. Williams ME, Tuttle KR. The next generation of diabetic nephropathy therapies: an update. Adv Chronic Kidney Dis 2005;12:212–22.

130. Bolton WK, Cattran DC, Williams ME, et al. ACTION I Investigator Group. Randomized trial of an

inhibitor of formation of advanced glycation end products in diabetic nephropathy. Am J Nephrol 2004;24:32–40.

131. Williams M, Bolton W, Khalifah R, et al. Effects of pyridoxamine in combined phase 2 studies of patients with type 1 and type 2 diabetes and overt nephropathy. Am J Nephrol 2007;27: 605–14.

132. Kanai Y, Lee WS, You G, et al. The human kidney low affinity Na+/glucose cotransporter SGLT2. Delineation of the major renal reabsorptive mechanism for D-glucose. J Clin Invest 1994;93:397–404.

133. Wright EM, Turk E. The sodium/glucose cotransport family SLC5. Pflugers Arch 2004;447(5):510–8.

134. Freitas HS, Anhê GF, Melo KF, et al. Na(+)-glucose transporter-2 messenger ribonucleic acid expression in kidney of diabetic rats correlates with glycemic levels: involvement of hepatocyte nuclear factor-1α expression and activity. Endocrinology 2008;149:717–24.

135. Rahmoune H, Thompson PW, Ward JM, et al. Glucose transporters in human renal proximal tubular cells isolated from the urine of patients with non insulin-dependent diabetes. Diabetes 2005;54:3427–34.

136. Nair S, Wilding JP. Sodium glucose cotransporter 2 inhibitors as a new treatment for diabetes mellitus. J Clin Endocrinol Metab 2010;95:34–42.

137. Bristol Myers-Squibb. Clinical trials disclosure: clinical trials for metabolic disease. Available at: http://ctr.bms.com/ctd/InitTrialAction.do?linkname= Metabolics&type=pharma&sortby. Accessed January 11, 2010.

The Role of Aldosteronism in Causing Obesity-Related Cardiovascular Risk

David A. Calhoun, MD[a],*, Kumar Sharma, MD[b]

KEYWORDS
- Aldosterone • Obesity • Hypertension • Adipocyte
- Spironolactone • Eplerenone

Obesity is strongly associated with an increased risk of cardiorenal disease, including hypertension, coronary artery disease, congestive heart failure, and chronic kidney disease (CKD). Recent studies indicate that hyperaldosteronism is a much more common cause of hypertension than had been thought. This observed increase in hyperaldosteronism has coincided with a worldwide increase in obesity, suggesting that these 2 disease processes may be mechanistically related. In this article, the role that aldosterone plays in mediating cardiovascular and renal disease risk is highlighted. In addition, the data linking adiposity to excess release of aldosterone are explored. Such data suggest that visceral adipose tissue serves as a source of potent stimuli of aldosteronogenesis, thereby implicating aldosterone as a potentially important mediator of obesity-related cardiovascular risk.

OBESITY AND HYPERTENSION

There is a direct correlation between increasing body weight and risk of hypertension. Data from the National Health and Nutrition Examination Survey 1999–2004 indicate that the prevalence of hypertension increases progressively with increasing body mass index (BMI, calculated as weight in kilograms divided by the square of height in meters) from about 15% among people with a BMI less than 25 kg/m^2 to approximately 40% among those with a BMI of 30 kg/m^2 or greater.[1] Analyses from the Framingham Heart Study suggest that approximately 78% of the risk of hypertension in men and 65% of that in women are directly related to excess body weight.[2] In some populations, there is an almost linear relation between increasing body weight and increasing severity of systolic and diastolic blood pressure.[3,4] The strong association between obesity and hypertension demonstrated in these and other studies suggests that obesity may be the most common cause of hypertension worldwide.

ALDOSTERONE AND HYPERTENSION

Cross-sectional and prospective studies indicate that aldosterone, independent of renin-angiotensin II, has an important contribution in the development and severity of hypertension. In a prospective analysis done as part of the ongoing Framingham Offspring Study, serum aldosterone, plasma renin concentration, and

Portions of this work were supported by the grant 5R01DK053867 from National Institute of Diabetes and Digestive and Kidney Diseases (K.S.).

[a] Vascular Biology and Hypertension Program, University of Alabama at Birmingham, 430 Biomedical Research Building II, 1530 3rd Avenue South, Birmingham, AL 35294-2180, USA
[b] Center for Renal Translational Medicine, University of California at San Diego/VA Medical System, Stein Building 4th Floor, 9500 Gilman Drive, MC 0711, La Jolla, CA 92093-0711, USA
* Corresponding author.
E-mail address: dcalhoun@uab.edu

the aldosterone/plasma renin ratio (ARR) were prospectively related to development of hypertension or to blood pressure progression (increase in severity).[5] In this evaluation of more than 3000 normotensive subjects who were followed for an average of 3 years, rates of incident hypertension and blood pressure progression rose across tertiles of increasing aldosterone levels, whereas the relation to renin was the opposite, with incident hypertension and blood pressure progression rising across tertiles of decreasing renin concentration (**Fig. 1**). The ARR was a stronger predictor of increasing blood pressure than aldosterone or renin alone, with the highest ARR quartile associated with a more than 2-fold risk of incident hypertension or blood pressure progression compared with the lowest quartile. These results strongly suggest that increasing aldosterone levels have an important contribution in the development of hypertension; this is particularly

true when aldosterone is in physiologic excess as suggested by suppressed renin levels.

Cross-sectional studies demonstrate a significant correlation between plasma aldosterone levels and untreated 24-hour ambulatory blood pressure levels. In an evaluation of African American and white French Canadian subjects, supine and standing plasma aldosterone levels were significantly related to daytime and nighttime systolic and diastolic blood pressure levels in the African American subjects.[6,7] In the white French Canadian subjects, standing aldosterone levels correlated with daytime and nighttime blood pressure, whereas supine aldosterone levels significantly related to nighttime systolic blood pressure. In both ethnic groups, blood pressure levels were unrelated to plasma renin activity (PRA), suggesting that aldosterone, more than the renin-angiotensin II axis, contributed to the severity of hypertension.

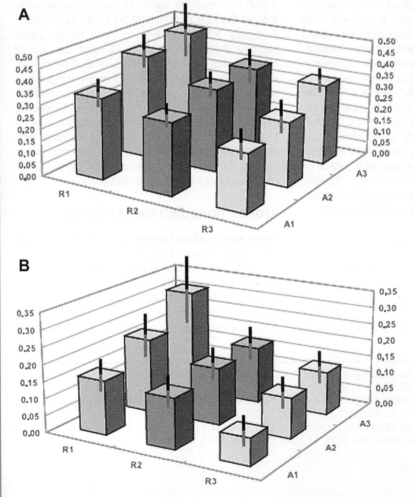

Fig. 1. Rates of blood pressure progression and incident hypertension among nonhypertensive participants. Age- and sex-adjusted incidence rates of blood pressure progression (*A*) and incident hypertension (*B*) at a mean of 3 years are shown across tertiles of aldosterone (A1–A3, first to third tertiles) and renin (R1–R3, first to third tertiles). Graded continuous increases in the risk of blood pressure progression and incident hypertension are found across increasing aldosterone and decreasing renin tertiles. Shaded and black error bars represent lower and upper 95% confidence bounds. (*From* Newton-Cheh C, Guo CY, Gona P, et al. Clinical and genetic correlates of aldosterone-to-renin ratio and relations to blood pressure in a community sample. Hypertension 2007;49:853; with permission.)

In a recent cross-sectional evaluation of 283 older adult subjects with and without a history of hypertension, there were significant correlations between systolic blood pressure and levels of plasma aldosterone following suppression with dexamethasone and after stimulation with corticotropin.[8] Diastolic blood pressure levels were significantly correlated with plasma aldosterone levels after dexamethasone administration. The associations were stronger in men than in women and remained after adjustment for potential confounding factors and after excluding subjects taking antihypertensive medications. In this analysis, there was an approximate 10 mm Hg difference in systolic pressure when subjects in the lowest and highest tertiles of aldosterone were compared.

These results of these observational studies and the prospective findings of the Framingham Offspring Study provide compelling evidence of the broad role of aldosterone in contributing to the onset and severity of hypertension in men and women. Aldosterone as an important mediator of hypertension is further supported by the general antihypertensive benefit of aldosterone blockade. For example, studies leading to the approval of eplerenone, a selective mineralocorticoid receptor (MR) antagonist, for the treatment of hypertension demonstrated broad efficacy in general hypertensive cohorts. In a prospective evaluation of 417 patients with mild to moderate hypertension, it was found that eplerenone reduced clinic blood pressure by up to 15.9 mm Hg.[9] These patients represented a generalized hypertensive cohort that was otherwise unselected, that is, patients were not screened based on aldosterone level, renin activity, or aldosterone/renin ratio. These results support the important role of aldosterone in contributing to the development of hypertension in a general population.

Historically, primary aldosteronism (PA) was reported to be an uncommon cause of hypertension with a prevalence of less than 1% among general hypertensive patients. However, with reports from investigators in Brisbane, Australia, from the early 1990s, the prevalence of PA has been described by clinics worldwide to be considerably higher, occurring in perhaps 5% to 10% of hypertensive patients.[10,11] Perhaps the most compelling of these is the PA Prevalence in Hypertensives (PAPY) study.[12] The study is particularly impressive in its prospective design, large sample size, and rigorous assessment of aldosterone status, including adrenal vein sampling of most patients with confirmed PA, and adrenalectomy when appropriate, thus allowing for definitive discrimination of idiopathic bilateral hyperplasia from an aldosterone-producing adenoma.

In the PAPY study, 1125 Italians who were newly diagnosed with hypertension agreed to be screened for PA, and the study included, whether biochemical PA was confirmed, lateralization studies (either adrenal vein sampling or adrenocortical scintigraphy), and adrenalectomy. Primary hyperaldosteronism was confirmed based on a high baseline ARR and high ARR after captopril suppression testing or with application of a previously validated logistic function. Aldosterone-producing adenomas were then confirmed by positive lateralization, surgical resection, pathologic examination, and clinical outcome after adrenalectomy. Subjects with confirmed primary hyperaldosteronism but without confirmed adrenal adenomas were diagnosed as having idiopathic PA.

Overall, the prevalence of biochemical PA was 11.2%. Approximately 43% of these cases could be attributed to an aldosterone-producing adenoma, with the remaining 57% considered to have an idiopathic cause. Accordingly, in this cohort of newly diagnosed hypertensive patients, the overall prevalence of PA secondary to an adrenal adenoma was 4.8%, and the prevalence of idiopathic PA was 6.4%. These results confirmed, through a prospective, scientifically rigorous evaluation, a now large body of evidence that indicates a high prevalence of PA in general hypertensive cohorts.

PA is especially common in patients with resistant hypertension. In an evaluation conducted at the University of Alabama at Birmingham, 20% of consecutive patients referred for resistant hypertension were diagnosed with PA.[13] A similarly high occurrence of PA in patients with resistant or poorly controlled hypertension was observed in separate prospective investigations by investigators in Seattle, Washington[14]; Oslo, Norway[15]; and Prague, Czech Republic,[16] suggesting that aldosterone excess commonly underlies resistance to antihypertensive treatment.

Recent study results suggest that, at least in patients with resistant hypertension, aldosterone also contributes to underlying hypertension beyond the approximately 20% of patients with classic PA. In a prospective evaluation of more than 250 patients with resistant hypertension, the authors found that even the subgroup of patients with normal or low aldosterone levels had evidence of greater intravascular fluid retention, as shown by higher levels of brain and atrial natriuretic peptide levels (**Fig. 2**).[17] The role of aldosterone in contributing broadly to resistance to antihypertensive treatment is further supported by the antihypertensive benefit of spironolactone in treating resistant hypertension. The authors and other investigators have found that spironolactone is effective in

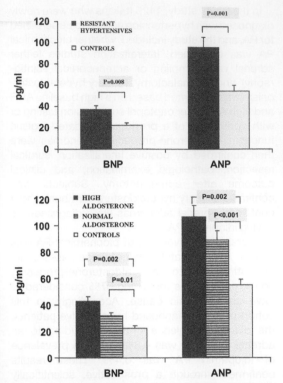

Fig. 2. Atrial natriuretic peptide (ANP) and brain natriuretic peptide (BNP) values in resistant hypertensive subjects and control (*top*). There was a significant incremental increase in ANP and BNP values among controls, resistant hypertensive subjects with normal status, and those with high aldosterone status (*bottom*). (*Adapted from* Gaddam KK, Nishizaka MK, Pratt-Ubunama MN, et al. Characterization of resistant hypertension: association between resistant hypertension, aldosterone, and persistent intravascular volume expansion. Arch Intern Med 2008;168:1161; with permission.)

treating resistant hypertension and that the degree of antihypertensive benefit is similar in patients with and without demonstrable hyperaldosteronism.[18] This broad benefit of spironolactone suggests that the role of aldosterone in causing hypertension in this group of patients is not limited to those with obvious aldosterone excess.

ALDOSTERONE AND CARDIORENAL DISEASE

A growing body of evidence links aldosterone excess to the development and progression of several cardiovascular disease processes separate from hypertension, including congestive heart failure, CKD, coronary artery disease, and stroke. In congestive heart failure, higher plasma aldosterone and angiotensin II levels predict increased

mortality. Cross-sectional studies implicate aldosterone excess as a probable contributor to the development of CKD. In an evaluation of 2700 participants in the Framingham Cohort Study, urinary sodium excretion was a strong positive predictor of urinary albumin excretion.[19] In addition, the top quintile of serum aldosterone levels was associated with a 21% higher urinary albumin excretion than the lowest quintile. In a separate study, patients with confirmed PA had significantly higher urinary albumin excretion compared with subjects with primary hypertension.[20] Other clinical studies have shown that chronic aldosterone excess is associated with increased left ventricular hypertrophy, greater diastolic dysfunction, exacerbation of endothelial dysfunction, and, recently, increased risk of various components of the metabolic syndrome.[21]

Consistent with these negative effects on cardiovascular risk factors, observational studies suggest that PA is associated with a rate of cardiovascular complications that seems to exceed that of primary hypertension. In one such comparison, patients diagnosed with PA were more than 4 times as likely to have had a stroke, 6.5 times as likely to have had a myocardial infarction, and more than 12 times as likely to have developed atrial fibrillation than general hypertensive patients matched as much as possible for duration and severity of hypertension.[22]

Prospective studies likewise link aldosterone to worse outcomes, whereas studies of aldosterone blockade demonstrate improvement in cardiovascular risk. Beygui and colleagues[23] reported that plasma aldosterone levels measured soon after admission predict cardiovascular morbidity and mortality and, in patients presenting with acute ST elevation, myocardial infarction. Patients in the highest quartile of plasma aldosterone level had a more than 2-fold increase in 6-month mortality compared with patients with lower aldosterone levels, as well as significantly more postinfarction cardiovascular complications including ventricular fibrillation, resuscitated cardiac arrest, and new or worsening congestive heart failure.

Aldosterone antagonists, even when added to renin-angiotensin blockers, reduce proteinuria in patients with CKD.[24] With respect to heart failure, the Randomized Aldactone Evaluation Study indicated that addition of low-dose spironolactone to regimens that included an angiotensin-converting enzyme (ACE) inhibitor in most patients significantly improved survival by 30%.[25] In the Eplerenone Post–Acute Myocardial Infarction Heart Failure Efficacy and Survival Study (EPHESUS), eplerenone added to an ACE inhibitor or angiotensin receptor blocker and β-blocker improved survival by 31% in patients with left ventricular dysfunction after acute myocardial infarction.[26] In showing benefit by directly blocking the MR, these intervention studies lend support to the role of aldosterone in directly contributing to development and/or progression of cardiorenal disease.

POTENTIAL MECHANISMS OF ALDOSTERONE-INDUCED END-ORGAN DAMAGE

A large body of experimental evidence has demonstrated that aldosterone excess in combination with high dietary salt intake induces perivascular inflammation and fibrosis.[27] These effects occur in multiple organs, including the heart, kidney, and brain. In addition, human studies suggest a variety of other effects presumed to negatively affect cardiovascular risk, including suppression of nitric oxide activity, impairment of endothelial function, and stimulation of thrombogenic pathways.[28]

Aldosterone receptors are classically localized to the principal cells of the cortical collecting duct, colonic epithelia, and salivary glands.[29] Aldosterone stimulates sodium reabsorption and potassium secretion via its binding to the intracellular MR. Aldosterone uses short-term and delayed transcriptional effects to stimulate the activity and synthesis of the epithelial sodium channel (ENaC) and sodium, potassium adenosine triphosphatase (Na,K-ATPase). The delayed stimulation of ENaC and the Na,K-ATPase is primarily caused by nuclear translocation of the ligand-receptor complex and binding to coregulators that stimulate gene transcription of ENaC (a subunit) and the Na,K-ATPase. The MR may form homodimers with itself and heterodimers with the glucocorticoid receptor. Cortisol may also bind the MR with great avidity; however, in protected sites, the presence of the cortisol-degrading enzyme 11-β-hydroxysteroid dehydrogenase-2 (11β-HSD2) prevents cortisol activation of the MR. A variety of coactivators that bind to the MR in the presence of aldosterone has been identified, including p160 family coactivators, steroid receptor coactivator 1 (SRC-1), SRC-2, and SRC-3, activating signal cointegrator 2 and peroxisome proliferator–activated receptor γ coactivator 1α.[30]

Aldosterone also stimulates ENaC activity via indirect effects that occur before the direct transcriptional stimulation of ENaC.[31] Aldosterone can stimulate rapid transcription of the serum- and glucocorticoid-induced kinase (SGK1). SGK1 phosphorylates the ubiquitin-protein ligase

Nedd4-2 at serine 328 and serine 212. In the absence of serine phosphorylation by SGK1, Nedd4-2 interacts with ENaC and induces ubiquitination and degradation of ENaC. When SGK1 phosphorylates ENaC, Nedd4-2 binds to 14-3-3 proteins, which interferes with its interaction with ENaC.[32] Thus, ENaC is then active for sodium transport. The increased sodium transport activity will lead to a net electronegative luminal voltage that drives H^+ secretion or K^+ secretion. Thus, the classic pattern of hypertension (associated with increased sodium uptake), metabolic alkalosis (increased H^+ secretion), and hypokalemia (increased K^+ secretion) results in patients with PA. Aldosterone in combination with salt loading can induce proteinuria, mesangial matrix accumulation, and tubulointerstitial fibrosis.[33] As noted earlier, increased sodium reabsorption could exacerbate proteinuria. Chronic hypokalemia may also result in interstitial fibrosis, possibly as a result of stimulation of renin release and transforming growth factor β (TGF-β) production.[34]

The MR has now been identified in a variety of other cell types, such as cardiac and vascular smooth muscle cells, and has been shown to mediate other functions of the MR, leading to inflammation, fibrosis, and metabolic regulation in cardiac and vascular tissue.[29] Recently, it has been found that glucocorticoids may regulate adipocyte differentiation via the MR in adipocytes. Because adipocytes have low levels of 11β-HSD2, the high levels of intracellular cortisol will not be degraded in adipocytes and can bind to and activate the MR. Thus, potentially, MR blockade may be beneficial in inhibiting adipocyte growth. The MR may mediate inflammation in multiple cell types via activation of NADPH oxidase.[35]

Aldosterone receptors have also been found in podocytes, mesangial cells, and fibroblasts.[36] Via the MR, aldosterone has been found to stimulate reactive oxygen species production, TGF-β production, and matrix synthesis in renal cells, leading to direct effects to stimulate inflammation and fibrosis. A recent study suggests that there may be local aldosterone production in the kidney itself, because adrenalectomized rats may have low levels of circulating aldosterone that seems to be produced from the kidney and possibly other sites.[37]

In recent studies, there seems to be a link between ENaC and the sodium retention noted with proteinuric and nephrotic states.[38] Increased filtration of circulating plasminogen enters the urine in states of heavy proteinuria. The plasminogen can be cleaved to plasmin in the urinary lumen via tubular urokinase-type plasminogen activator. The active plasmin is then free to cleave the luminal facing ENaC, thus activating it and allowing for excess sodium reabsorption. Although a luminal diuretic such amiloride or triamterene may be the preferred way to block the enhanced ENaC activity, presumably aldosterone receptor blockade may also limit the degree of ENaC channels entering the lumen and be useful in proteinuric states.

OBESITY AND ALDOSTERONE

The cause of the apparent increase in aldosterone excess and its role in contributing to the development of hypertension over the last several decades remain unexplained. Demonstration of this growing role of aldosterone in mediating hypertension and other cardiovascular complications has coincided with a progressive increase in worldwide rates of obesity, suggesting a possible causative relation between increasing body weight and stimulation of aldosterone release. Population-based observational studies suggest a correlation between obesity and aldosterone levels, whereas experimental studies implicate adipocyte-related factors as possible stimuli of aldosterone release. If adiposity is confirmed to either directly or indirectly stimulate aldosterone release, it would serve to mechanistically link obesity-related hypertension to excess aldosterone. This link would represent an important clinical advance in explaining underlying mechanisms of obesity-induced hypertension and would support the preferential use of aldosterone antagonists to treat prehypertension and hypertension in obese patients.

Several cross-sectional studies have demonstrated a significant relation between aldosterone levels and indexes of obesity, including BMI and waist circumference. In one of the earliest studies linking aldosterone to obesity, Rocchini and colleagues[39] evaluated 30 obese and 10 nonobese adolescents before and after weight loss. The obese adolescents had significantly higher supine and 2-hour upright plasma aldosterone concentrations. Compared with an obese control group who had maintained their body weight, weight loss resulted in a significant decrease in plasma aldosterone level without a decrease in PRA. In addition to weight loss being associated with a significant decrease in blood pressure, there was a significant correlation between the change in plasma aldosterone level and the change in mean blood pressure. Although a small study, these findings were significant in demonstrating that obese adolescents have higher plasma aldosterone levels than nonobese adolescents, that aldosterone decreased with weight loss seemingly

independent of renin activity, and that the decrease in aldosterone levels correlated with decrease in blood pressure. These findings support obesity-related increases in blood pressure being attributable, at least in part, to excess aldosterone independent of renin-angiotensin stimulation.

In another early study, Goodfriend and colleagues[40] measured visceral adipose tissue by computed tomography, total fat mass by dual energy x-ray absorptiometry, and plasma aldosterone levels in 28 normotensive women and 27 normotensive men. Plasma aldosterone levels in women correlated directly with visceral adipose tissue independent of PRA. There were no corresponding correlations in men. Seventeen women and 15 men completed a weight reduction regimen, losing an average of 15.1 ± 1.2 kg. After weight loss, plasma aldosterone level was significantly lower; however, the correlations of aldosterone with visceral adipose tissue in women persisted. In the female subjects, blood pressure correlated with plasma aldosterone level before and after weight loss. In a separate analysis of a largely male cohort, similar correlations were observed between aldosterone levels and measurements of visceral adipose tissue.[41] These results link adiposity, particularly visceral adiposity, to aldosterone release, which then relates to blood pressure levels.

In a cross-sectional analysis, Andronico and colleagues[42] found that 39 severely obese subjects (mean BMI 47.8 ± 1.4 kg/m^2) being screened for bariatric surgery had significantly higher plasma aldosterone levels and a higher mean aldosterone/PRA ratio than lean (mean BMI of 24.1 ± 0.4) and mildly obese (mean BMI 31.5 ± 0.9 kg/m^2) control subjects. PRA values were higher in the severely obese controls compared with mildly obese controls but not the lean controls, suggesting that the greater aldosterone levels were not attributable solely to renin-angiotensin activation.

As observed initially by Goodfriend and colleagues,[40] the positive relation between adiposity and aldosterone may be most consistent in women. In an evaluation of 109 hypertensive African American subjects and 73 hypertensive white French Canadians, El-Gharbawy and colleagues[6] found significant associations between aldosterone and obesity in women but not in men. In particular, among African American women, supine plasma aldosterone level was significantly correlated with BMI, body surface area, and hip circumference, but not with waist-to-hip ratio or percent body fat as determined from measurements of skinfold thickness. There were no significant correlations of plasma aldosterone level with any of the anthropomorphic measurements in African American men or in French Canadian women and men.

A subsequent analysis of 466 African Americans that included an equal proportion of normotensive and hypertensive subjects was done by the same laboratory.[43] Overall, systolic blood pressure positively correlated with BMI and plasma aldosterone level and inversely with PRA. Plasma aldosterone level was significantly correlated with waist circumference but not with BMI. Among hypertensive subjects, plasma aldosterone levels were significantly higher and PRA was significantly lower with increasing BMI strata. The investigators concluded that their findings suggested that in African Americans, hypertension related to visceral obesity may be mediated by aldosterone.

Evaluation of 2 large Italian cohorts have also reported that plasma aldosterone levels correlate with indices of adiposity. Mulè and colleagues[44] prospectively evaluated 450 subjects referred to their hypertension center. Antihypertensive medications, if present, were withdrawn for 2 weeks before evaluation. By univariate analysis, plasma aldosterone level was significantly correlated with BMI and waist circumference. The correlations remained significant even after multivariate adjustments. In this same evaluation, plasma aldosterone levels were also positively correlated with 24-hour ambulatory systolic and diastolic blood pressure, as well as indices of left ventricular mass as measured by echocardiography. Overall, these results suggest that obesity is associated with increased aldosterone levels, which may then independently contribute to higher blood pressure levels and greater left ventricular mass. These results are important in linking aldosterone to cardiovascular complications of obesity, specifically high blood pressure and left ventricular hypertrophy.

Evaluation of the PAPY cohort by Rossi and colleagues[45] also indicated a significant correlation between plasma aldosterone level and BMI. The analysis included the 1125 subjects prospectively enrolled in the PAPY study, 999 of whom were diagnosed with primary hypertension and 126 with PA. Plasma aldosterone level was positively correlated with BMI in the cohort of patients with primary hypertension, with the correlation being strongest in the most overweight subjects. In subjects with confirmed PA, plasma aldosterone levels were not correlated with BMI. These results suggest that in the absence of PA, that is, in patients with presumed primary hypertension, obesity seems to be an important mediator of aldosterone secretion consistent with a pathophysiological link between fat disposition and the synthesis and/or secretion of aldosterone. In patients with classic PA, this link is not evident, suggesting an autonomous release of aldosteronism independent of adiposity.

Consistent with observational studies linking aldosterone to obesity, weight loss studies support a mechanistic link between adipocytes and aldosterone release. In the studies of Rocchini and colleagues[39] and Goodfriend and colleagues,[40] weight loss was associated with significant decreases in plasma aldosterone levels. In the former study, the decrease in aldosterone was reported to occur independent of changes in PRA. Tuck and colleagues[46] had likewise reported in an earlier study that successful weight loss in obese subjects is associated with significant decreases in plasma aldosterone levels. In this study, the decrease in aldosterone level was also accompanied by significant decreases in PRA, suggesting that obesity may be associated with a generalized stimulation of the renin-angiotensin-aldosterone system. These results are consistent with 2 recent studies relating weight loss to reductions in renin-angiotensin-aldosterone activation. In the first study, Engeli and colleagues[47] reported that an approximate 5% weight loss in obese women was associated with significant reductions in circulating angiotensinogen, renin, and aldosterone levels, as well as significant reduction in angiotensinogen expression in adipose tissue biopsy samples. In the second study, Dall'Asta and colleagues[48] found that weight loss following laparoscopic banding in severely obese subjects is associated with decreases in plasma aldosterone levels and PRA. Overall, these studies, although individually small, provide interventional confirmation that obesity contributes to increased aldosterone release.

Recent studies of patients infected with human immunodeficiency virus (HIV) provide intriguing support that visceral adiposity contributes to hyperaldosteronism. HIV infection is sometimes associated with abnormal deposition of visceral fat. In one recent analysis, approximately 22% of subjects infected with HIV had significant abdominal lipohypertrophy.[49] In a separate evaluation, Lo and colleagues[50] found that women with increased visceral abdominal tissue infected with HIV had higher aldosterone levels compared with age- and BMI-matched healthy controls and women without visceral fat accumulation with HIV infection. In the HIV-infected patients with increased visceral fat accumulation, the 24-hour aldosterone secretion was positively correlated with BMI and the amount of visceral fat tissue. These results provide further support that excess abdominal adiposity has an important contribution in inappropriate secretion of aldosterone.

A positive correlation between aldosterone and adiposity has not been universally observed. In a large and rigorous evaluation of 1172 subjects in the United Kingdom, Alvarez-Madrazo and colleagues[51] did not find that plasma aldosterone levels correlated with BMI. This observation was true for the entire cohort and also a smaller subgroup of subjects who were not receiving any antihypertensive medications. In fact, the aldosterone/renin ratio was negatively correlated with BMI, whereas the plasma renin concentration was positively correlated. Unlike the other studies discussed earlier, the investigators did not find evidence that obesity was associated with increased aldosterone levels. At this point, there is no obvious explanation for these negative results and the multiple positive results discussed earlier.

OBESITY AND BLOOD PRESSURE RESPONSE TO ALDOSTERONE BLOCKADE

If obesity contributes to aldosterone excess, it would be anticipated that aldosterone antagonists would be more effective in lowering blood pressure in obese subjects than in nonobese subjects. Although there is little, if any, direct data assessing this possibility, preliminary data suggestive of a preferential benefit of aldosterone blockade in relation to adiposity are emerging. In a retrospective analysis of the blood pressure response of spironolactone in patients with CKD, Khosla and colleagues[52] found that the largest blood pressure response was observed in obese African American women. In a recent prospective assessment of the antihypertensive efficacy of spironolactone in patients with resistant hypertension, de Souza and colleagues[53] found that a higher waist circumference predicted a more favorable blood pressure response.

Although these studies are provocative, well-designed clinical trials specifically evaluating the antihypertensive efficacy of aldosterone antagonists in obese patients are clearly needed to test for enhanced benefit. If such studies confirm that aldosterone antagonists are more effective in obese than in nonobese patients, it would provide important supporting data for the role of adipose tissue in causing hyperaldosteronism and would provide rationale for preferential use of aldosterone antagonists in obese hypertensive and, perhaps, prehypertensive patients.

POTENTIAL MECHANISMS OF ADIPOCYTE-DERIVED HYPERALDOSTERONISM

Potential mechanisms by which adipocytes may contribute to excess aldosterone secretion include generalized stimulation of the renin-angiotensin-aldosterone system and, separately, release from adipocytes of secretagogues specific for aldosterone. Adipocytes appear to have all the components of the renin-angiotensin system (RAS) and thus may produce locally generated angiotensin II.[54–56] As noted earlier, adipocytes may also produce aldosterone and thus may directly contribute to systemic aldosterone levels. A generalized stimulation of the renin-angiotensin-aldosterone system is supported by weight loss studies that demonstrate reductions in components of the pathway, including aldosterone.[48] In addition to this generalized effect, a growing body of evidence suggests that adipokines, adipocytes release factors, may stimulate aldosterone release independent of renin-angiotensin.[57]

Obesity is associated with increased oxidative stress and circulating levels of free fatty acids, of which the most readily oxidized are the polyunsaturated acids, and, in particular, linoleic acid, which may be the most abundant. Goodfriend and colleagues[58] have shown that oxidized derivatives of linoleic acid stimulate release of aldosterone from isolated rat adrenal cells, with one specific derivative, 12,13-epoxy-9-keto-10(trans)-octadecenoic acid, being particularly potent. These studies suggest that adipocytes release free fatty acids that, once oxidized in the liver, serve as potent stimuli of aldosteronogenesis independent of angiotensin II.

Ehrhart-Bornstein and colleagues[59] have also provided evidence of adipocyte secretory products that directly stimulate adrenocortical aldosterone secretion. In their study, placing human adrenocortical cells in a medium exposed to isolated adipocytes resulted in a 7-fold increase in aldosterone secretion. This stimulatory effect was not blocked by valsartan, an angiotensin receptor blocker, indicating an effect independent of angiotensin II. Subsequent studies by this same laboratory have demonstrated that human adipocytes induce an extracellularly regulated kinase (ERK) 1 or ERK2 mitogen-activated protein kinase–mediated upregulation of steroidogenic acute regulatory protein and an associated angiotensin II sensitization of human adrenocortical cells.[60]

In an experiment with obese diabetic rats, Jeon and colleagues[57] demonstrated that C1q TNF-related protein 1 (CTRP1), a member of the CTRP superfamily, may also function as a potent, aldosterone-stimulating factor. The investigators reported that CTRP1, which is expressed at high levels in adipose tissue and in the zona glomerulosa of the adrenal cortex, the site of aldosterone production, induces a dose-dependent increase in aldosterone production and that angiotensin II–induced aldosterone release is mediated by stimulation of CTRP1 secretion. These pathophysiologic studies linking visceral adiposity to aldosterone secretion provide mechanistic support for the hypothesis that obesity contributes directly to inappropriate release of aldosterone, resulting in a state of relative aldosterone excess.

SUMMARY

Obesity and aldosterone excess are common. Observational studies indicate that indices of adiposity such as BMI, waist circumference, and measure of visceral tissue correlate with aldosterone levels. In vitro studies suggest that adipocytes release factors that stimulate aldosterone secretion independent of renin-angiotensin II. These studies support the concept that obesity contributes to hyperaldosteronism. Aldosterone excess has been shown to have an important contribution in the development and progression of cardiovascular disease, particularly hypertension. Therefore, confirming that obesity contributes to the development of hyperaldosteronism would have several important clinical implications. First, it would implicate aldosterone as an important mediator of cardiovascular risk in obese patients. Second, it would support preferential use of aldosterone antagonists to treat hypertension in obese patients, and, more broadly, to minimize risk of cardiovascular complications. At present, there is convincing data that inhibitors of the aldosterone receptor or the aldosterone-stimulated ENaC channel is associated with impressive reductions in sodium retention and blood pressure in patients with obesity and proteinuria. Furthermore, patients with CKD and obesity may also have preferential benefits from inhibitors of the aldosterone receptor to block ongoing renal fibrosis. However, the relative benefit of aldosterone and ENaC blockers versus inhibitors of the RAS are unclear. Given the large amount of data supporting the cardioprotective and renoprotective effects of the RAS inhibitors, it is likely prudent to use RAS inhibitors as first-line agents and consider aldosterone blockers as second- or third-line agents, depending on the parameters of proteinuria, electrolyte levels, sodium retention, and underlying cardiovascular status. Before such use can be routinely recommended, outcome studies testing these proposed benefits are needed.

REFERENCES

1. Ong KL, Cheung BM, Man YB, et al. Prevalence, awareness, treatment, and control of hypertension among United States Adults 1999–2004. Hypertension 2007;49:69–75.

2. Garrison RJ, Kannel WB, Stokes J III, et al. Incidence and precursors of hypertension in young adults: the Framingham Off-spring Study. Prev Med 1987;16:235–51.

3. Sharabi Y, Gotto I, Huerta M, et al. Susceptibility of the influence of weight on blood pressure in men versus women: lessons from a large-scale study of adults. Am J Hypertens 2004;17:404–8.

4. Jones DW, Kim JS, Andrew ME, et al. Body mass index and blood pressure in Korean men and women: the Korean National Blood Pressure Survey. J Hypertens 1994;12:1433–7.

5. Newton-Cheh C, Guo CY, Gona P, et al. Clinical and genetic correlates of aldosterone-to-renin ratio and relations to blood pressure in a community sample. Hypertension 2007;49:846–56.

6. El-Gharbawy AH, Nadig VS, Kotchen JM, et al. Arterial pressure, left ventricular mass, and aldosterone in essential hypertension. Hypertension 2001;37:845–50.

7. Grim CE, Cowley AW, Hamet P, et al. Hyperaldosteronism and hypertension: ethnic differences. Hypertension 2005;45:766–72.

8. Reynolds RM, Walker BR, Phillips DI, et al. Programming of hypertension: associations of plasma aldosterone in adult men and women with birthweight, cortisol, and blood pressure. Hypertension 2009;53:932–6.

9. Weinbereger MH, Roniker B, Krause SL, et al. Eplerenone, a selective aldosterone blocker, in mild-to-moderate hypertension. Am J Hypertens 2002;15:709–16.

10. Gordon RD, Ziesak MD, Tunny TJ, et al. Evidence that primary aldosteronism may not be uncommon: 12% incidence among antihypertensive drug trail volunteers. Clin Exp Pharmacol Physiol 1993;20:296–8.

11. Gordon RD, Stowasser M, Tunyy TJ, et al. High incidence of primary aldosteronism in 199 patients referred with hypertension. Clin Exp Pharmacol Physiol 1994;21:315–8.

12. Rossi GP, Bernini G, Caliumi C, et al. PAPY Study Investigators. A prospective study of the prevalence of primary aldosteronism in 1,125 hypertensive patients. J Am Coll Cardiol 2006;48:2293–300.

13. Calhoun DA, Nishizaka MK, Zaman MA, et al. High prevalence of primary aldosteronism among black and white subjects with resistant hypertension. Hypertension 2002;40:892–6.

14. Gallay BJ, Ahmad S, Xu L, et al. Screening for primary aldosteronism without discontinuing hypertensive medications: plasma aldosterone-renin ratio. Am J Kidney Dis 2001;37:699–705.

15. Eide IK, Torjesen PA, Drolsum A, et al. Low-renin status in therapy-resistant hypertension: a clue to efficient treatment. J Hypertens 2004;22:2217–26.

16. Štrauch B, Zelinka T, Hampf M, et al. Prevalence of primary hyperaldosteronism in moderate to severe hypertension in the Central Europe region. J Hum Hypertens 2003;17:349–52.

17. Gaddam KK, Nishizaka MK, Pratt-Ubunama MN, et al. Resistant hypertension characterized by increased aldosterone levels and persistent intravascular volume expansion. Arch Intern Med 2008; 168:1159–64.

18. Nishizaka MK, Zaman MA, Calhoun DA. Efficacy of low-dose spironolactone in subjects with resistant hypertension. Am J Hypertens 2003;16:925–30.

19. Fox CS, Larson MG, Hwang SJ, et al. Cross-sectional relations of serum aldosterone and urine sodium excretion to urinary albumin excretion in a community-based sample. Kidney Int 2006;69:2064–9.

20. Rossi GP, Bernini G, Giovambattista D, et al. PAPY Study Investigators. Renal damage in primary aldosteronism: results of the PAPY Study. Hypertension 2006;48:232–8.

21. Bochud M, Nussberger J, Bovet P, et al. Plasma aldosterone is independently associated with the metabolic syndrome. Hypertension 2006;48:239–45.

22. Milliez P, Girerd X, Plouin PF, et al. Evidence of an increased rate of cardiovascular events in patients with primary aldosteronism. J Am Coll Cardiol 2005;45:1243–8.

23. Beygui F, Collet JP, Benoliel JJ, et al. High plasma aldosterone levels on admission are associated with death in patient presenting with acute ST-elevation myocardial infarction. Circulation 2006;114: 2604–10.

24. Epstein M, Williams GH, Weinberger M, et al. Selective aldosterone blockade with eplerenone reduces albuminuria in patients with type 2 diabetes. Clin J Am Soc Nephrol 2006;1:940–51.

25. Pitt B, Zannad F, Remme WJ, et al. The effect of spironolactone on morbidity and mortality in patients with severe heart failure. Randomized Aldactone Evaluation Study Investigators. N Engl J Med 1999;341:709–17.

26. Pitt B, Remme W, Zannad F, et al. Eplerenone, a selective aldosterone blocker, in patients with left ventricular dysfunction after myocardial infarction. N Engl J Med 2003;348:1309–21.

27. Rocha R, Stier CT Jr, Kifor I, et al. Aldosterone: a mediator of myocardial necrosis and renal arteriopathy. Endocrinology 2000;141:3871–8.

28. Schiffrin EL. Effects of aldosterone on the vasculature. Hypertension 2006;47:312–8.

29. Zennaro MC, Caprio M, Feve B. Mineralocorticoid receptors in the metabolic syndrome. Trends Endocrinol Metab 2009;20:444–51.

30. Yokota K, Shibata H, Kurihara I, et al. Coactivation of the N-terminal transactivation of mineralocorticoid receptor by Ubc9. J Biol Chem 2007;282:1998–2010.

31. Flores SY, Loffing-Cueni D, et al. Aldosterone-induced serum and glucocorticoid-induced kinase 1 expression is accompanied by Nedd4-2 phosphorylation and increased Na^+ transport in cortical collecting duct cells. J Am Soc Nephrol 2005;16:2279–87.

32. Ichimura T, Yamamura H, Sasamoto K, et al. 14-3-3 proteins modulate the expression of epithelial $Na+$ channels by phosphorylation-dependent interaction with Nedd4-2 ubiquitin ligase. J Biol Chem 2005; 280:13187–94.

33. Kiyomoto H, Rafiq K, Mostofa M, et al. Possible underlying mechanisms responsible for aldosterone and mineralocorticoid receptor-dependent renal injury. J Pharmacol Sci 2008;108:399–405.

34. Ray PE, Suga S, Liu XH, et al. Chronic potassium depletion induces renal injury, salt sensitivity, and hypertension in young rats. Kidney Int 2001;59: 1850–8.

35. Nakamura T, Kataoka K, Fukuda M, et al. Critical role of apoptosis signal-regulating kinase 1 in aldosterone/salt-induced cardiac inflammation and fibrosis. Hypertension 2009;54:544–51.

36. Lee SH, Yoo TH, Nam BY, et al. Activation of local aldosterone system within podocytes is involved in apoptosis under diabetic conditions. Am J Physiol Renal Physiol 2009;297:F1381–90.

37. Xue C, Siragy HM. Local renal aldosterone system and its regulation by salt, diabetes, and angiotensin II type 1 receptor. Hypertension 2005;46:584–90.

38. Svenningsen P, Bistrup C, Friis UG, et al. Plasmin in nephrotic urine activates the epithelial sodium channel. J Am Soc Nephrol 2009;20:299–310.

39. Rocchini AP, Katch VL, Gerkin R, et al. Role of aldosterone in blood pressure regulation of obese adolescents. Am J Cardiol 1986;57:613–8.

40. Goodfriend TL, Kelley DE, Goodpaster BH, et al. Visceral obesity and insulin resistance are associated with plasma aldosterone levels in women. Obes Res 1999;7:355–62.

41. Goodfriend TL, Egan BM, Kelley DE. Plasma aldosterone, plasma lipoproteins, obesity and insulin in humans. Prostaglandins Leukot Essent Fatty Acids 1999;60:401–5.

42. Andronico G, Cottone S, Mangano MT, et al. Insulin, renin-aldosterone system and blood pressure in obese people. Int J Obes Relat Metab Disord 2001;25:239–42.

43. Kidambi S, Kotchen JM, Keishnaswami S, et al. Aldosterone contributes to blood pressure variance and to likelihood of hypertension in normal-weight and overweight African Americans. Am J Hypertens 2009;22:1303–8.

44. Mulè G, Nardi E, Cusimano P, et al. Plasma aldosterone and its relationships with left ventricular mass in essential hypertensive patients with metabolic syndrome. Am J Hypertens 2008;21:1055–61.

45. Rossi GP, Belfiore A, Bernini G, et al. Body moss index predicts plasma aldosterone concentrations in overweight-obese primary hypertensive patients. J Clin Endocrinol Metab 2008;93:2566–71.

46. Tuck ML, Sowers J, Dornfeld L, et al. The effect of weight reduction on blood pressure, plasma renin activity, and plasma aldosterone levels in obese patients. N Engl J Med 1981;304:930–3.

47. Engeli S, Böhnke J, Gorzelniak K, et al. Weight loss and the renin-angiotensin-aldosterone system. Hypertension 2005;45:356–62.

48. Dall'Asta C, Vedani P, Manunta P, et al. Effect of weight loss through laparoscopic gastric banding on blood pressure, plasma renin activity and aldosterone levels in morbid obesity. Nutr Metab Cardiovasc Dis 2009;19:110–4.

49. Nguyen A, Calmy A, Schiffer V, et al. Lipodystrophy and weight changes: data from the Swiss HIV Cohort Study, 2000–2006. HIV Med 2008;9:142–50.

50. Lo J, Looby ED, Wei J, et al. Increased aldosterone among HIV-infected women with visceral fat accumulation. AIDS 2009;23:2366–70.

51. Alvarez-Madrazo S, Padmanabhan S, Mayosi BM, et al. Familial and phenotypic associations of the aldosterone renin ratio. J Clin Endocrinol Metab 2009;94:4324–33.

52. Khosla N, Kalaitzidis R, Bakris GL. Predictors of hyperkalemia risk following hypertension control with aldosterone blockade. Am J Nephrol 2009;30:418–24.

53. de Souza F, Muxfeldt E, Fiszman R, et al. Efficacy of spironolactone therapy in patients with true resistant hypertension. Hypertension 2010;55:147–52.

54. Weiland F, Verspohl EJ. Local formation of angiotensin peptides with paracrine activity by adipocytes. J Pept Sci 2009;15:767–76.

55. Kershaw EE, Flier JS. Adipose tissue as an endocrine organ. J Clin Endocrinol Metab 2004;89:2548–56.

56. Engeli S, Schling P, Gorzelniak K, et al. The adipose-tissue renin-angiotensin-aldosterone system: role in the metabolic syndrome? Int J Biochem Cell Biol 2003;35:807–25.

57. Jeon JH, Kim KY, Kim J, et al. A novel adipokine CTRP1 stimulates aldosterone production. FASEB J 2008;22:1502–11.

58. Goodfriend TL, Ball DL, Egan BM, et al. Epoxy-keto derivative of linoleic acid stimulates aldosterone secretion. Hypertension 2004;43:358–63.

59. Ehrhart-Bornstein M, Lamounier-Zepter V, Schraven A, et al. Human adipocytes secrete mineralocorticoid-releasing factors. Proc Natl Acad Sci U S A 2003;100:14211–6.

60. Krug AW, Vleugels K, Schinner S, et al. Human adipocytes induce an ERK1/2 MAP kinases-mediated upregulation of steroidogenic acute regulatory protein (StAR) and angiotensin II-sensitization in human adrenocortical cells. Int J Obes (Lond) 2007;31:1605–16.

Early Intervention Strategies to Lower Cardiovascular Risk in Early Nephropathy: Focus on Dyslipidemia

Matthew J. Sorrentino, MD

KEYWORDS

- Dyslipidemia • Microalbuminuria
- Chronic kidney disease • Statins

It is estimated that nearly 20 million adults have chronic kidney disease (CKD) in the United States.[1] And yet, less than 2% of these individuals will progress to end stage renal disease. Most patients with CKD will die of a cardiovascular event long before they will require renal replacement therapy. The Hypertension Detection and Follow-up Program showed that an elevated serum creatinine is a potent independent risk factor for all-cause mortality and that the most frequent cause of death was a cardiovascular event rather than a renal cause.[2] The National Kidney Foundation Task Force on Cardiovascular Disease in Chronic Renal Disease highlighted the increased cardiovascular disease risk in patients with CKD and recommended that CKD should be considered a high-risk category for cardiovascular disease (CVD) risk stratification.[3] This designation would put patients with CKD in the coronary heart disease risk-equivalent category suggesting that CVD risk in patients with CKD is similar to individuals that already have documented heart disease or a previous myocardial infarction.

CARDIOVASCULAR RISK FACTORS

There is a high prevalence of atherosclerotic disease in patients with CKD. This prevalence is likely caused by the high prevalence of cardiovascular risk factors associated with CKD. It is important to identify these risk factors so that risk modifying treatments can be prescribed to improve the prognosis of patients with CKD. In addition to traditional cardiovascular risk factors, patients with CKD tend to accrue a large number of nontraditional risk factors that may further augment CVD risk (**Box 1**).

Traditional CVD risk factors are those factors that have been well defined and are independently associated with risk in the general population usually by large prospective cohort studies, such as the Framingham study. Traditional risk factors that tend to cluster in patients with CKD include older age, hypertension, diabetes mellitus, and a low high-density lipoprotein cholesterol. Total and low-density lipoprotein cholesterol are also correlated with mortality in patients with CKD, but there exists a U-shaped relationship that is most notable in patients with end stage renal disease.[4] The increased prevalence of malnutrition in this cohort of patients may help to explain the apparently paradoxic finding that hypocholesterolemia is a potent predictor of mortality in end stage renal disease.

The cardiovascular risk attributed to traditional risk factors in patients with CKD largely parallels the relationship described in the general population.[5] The National Cholesterol Education Program Adult Treatment Panel III report recommends using a risk factor algorithm based on the Framingham risk equation to calculate CVD risk.[6] The projected risk of CVD events for individuals with CKD

Section of Cardiology, Department of Medicine, University of Chicago Pritzker School of Medicine, 5841 South Maryland Avenue, MC 6080, Chicago, IL 60637, USA
E-mail address: msorrent@medicine.bsd.uchicago.edu

Cardiol Clin 28 (2010) 529–539
doi:10.1016/j.ccl.2010.04.009
0733-8651/10/$ – see front matter © 2010 Elsevier Inc. All rights reserved.

has been found to be similar or somewhat higher when compared with reference populations from the Framingham cohort.[7] The Framingham risk score, however, may be insufficient to capture the full extent of CVD risk in these patients because of the presence of nontraditional risk factors not represented by the risk score. In addition, individuals with CKD may have a longer and more severe exposure to certain risk factors, such as hypertension and diabetes, when compared with the general population evaluated in cohort studies.

Nontraditional risk factors are those factors that are related to CKD and CVD but not necessarily found to be strong independent factors in multiple regression analysis studies. To be considered a risk factor, the factor should have a biologic reason to promote CVD, increase with severity as renal function declines, demonstrate an association between the risk factor and CVD in patients with CKD, and ideally have clinical trial data that shows that targeting the factor can reduce CVD outcomes.[5] Many of the proposed risk factors have shown an association between the factor and CVD in observational studies in patients with CKD but have not yet been proven to be beneficial treatment targets in randomized studies.

Nontraditional risk factors include factors that have been associated with CVD in the general population and those that appear to be unique to patients with CKD. General population risk factors include additional lipid factors, such as lipoprotein (a), lipoprotein remnants, small dense LDL cholesterol, and abnormal apolipoproteins; inflammatory factors, such as CRP; and thrombotic factors, such as hyperhomocysteinemia. Renal-specific factors include albuminuria, anemia, excessive oxidative stress, and abnormal calcium/phosphate metabolism.

DYSLIPIDEMIA OF CHRONIC KIDNEY DISEASE

Multiple lipoprotein abnormalities have been described in patients with CKD. Common lipid profile patterns in patients with CKD with and without nephrotic range proteinuria are summarized in **Table 1**. In general, the prevalence of dyslipidemia in chronic kidney disease varies with the degree of renal insufficiency and the presence of proteinuria.[8] As glomerular filtration rate (GFR) declines, HDL cholesterol decreases and triglycerides increase. Nephrotic range proteinuria is associated with increased levels of total and LDL cholesterol, increased triglycerides, and decreased HDL cholesterol. The hyperlipidemia of the nephrotic syndrome is thought to be a consequence of increased lipoprotein synthesis in the liver in response to urinary loss of proteins and reduced oncotic pressure from hypoalbuminemia.

Diabetes is commonly associated with CKD and patients with diabetes likewise have a high prevalence of lipid abnormalities. Diabetics, especially those with poor glycemic control, have a similar dyslipidemic pattern to patients with CKD with elevated triglycerides and low HDL cholesterol. Higher triglyceride levels are associated with smaller and denser LDL particles.[9] Small, dense LDL particles are thought to be more atherogenic than larger particles. Smaller LDL particles are more likely to become oxidized, bind poorly to the LDL receptor, and have delayed clearance from the plasma.[10] These characteristics may help explain why patients with normal LDL

Table 1
Common lipid profiles in patients with CKD with or without nephritic proteinuria

Lipid Parameter	Nephrotic Range Proteinuria	Minimal Proteinuria
Total cholesterol	↑	↔ or ↓
LDL cholesterol	↑	↔, ↓ or ↑
Small, dense LDL	↑	↑
HDL cholesterol	↑	↓
Triglycerides	↑	↑
IDL cholesterol	↑	↑
ApoA-I, ApoA-II	↓	↓

Abbreviation: IDL, intermediate-density lipoprotein.
Data from Vaziri ND. Dyslipidemia of chronic renal failure: the nature, mechanisms, and potential consequences. Am J Physiol Renal Physiol 2006;290(2):F262–72.

cholesterol levels have increased cardiovascular risk if they predominantly have smaller and denser LDL particles.

Changes in apolipoproteins occur early in CKD and typically precede changes in lipid levels. Apolipoproteins A-I and A-II are the major lipoproteins associated with HDL particles. Reduced concentrations of apolipoprotein (Apo)A-I and ApoA-II are responsible for the low HDL-cholesterol levels. The lower apolipoprotein levels may be due, in part, to downregulation of hepatic ApoA-I gene expression[11] or a consequence of chronic inflammation leading to decreased albumin and HDL cholesterol levels.[12]

Plasma triglyceride levels are frequently elevated in patients with CKD. Triglyceride elevations are likely caused by increased plasma concentrations and impaired clearance of very low density lipoproteins (VLDL). Animal models suggest that low albumin is associated with reduced endothelial-bound lipoprotein lipase (LPL), the enzyme responsible for catabolism of triglycerides from lipoproteins.[13] Low LPL levels would lead to higher VLDL levels. In addition, animals with nephrotic syndrome have reduced binding of VLDL to LPL as a result of dysfunctional HDL particles. Therefore it appears that the high triglyceride levels are caused in part by low catabolism from reduced LPL levels and reduced lipoprotein binding to LPL, which leads to the accumulation of atherogenic VLDL remnants.[14] Finally, insulin resistance, which is frequently associated with renal insufficiency, may help promote increased production of VLDL particles by the liver. Furthermore, clearance of chylomicrons is also impaired and elevated levels of chylomicron remnants are seen in patients with CKD. Chylomicrons are triglyceride-rich particles. The elevated levels of remnant particles have been associated with an increased CVD risk.

MICROALBUMINURIA AND PROTEINURIA

Microalbuminuria is a small abnormal amount of protein in the urine usually defined as an albumin excretion of 30 to 300 mg/d. Albuminuria higher than 300 mg/d is considered overt proteinuria and is detectable by urinary dipstick. Spot urine specimens assessing the albumin/creatinine ratio (ACR) is an easy and quick method to screen for microalbuminuria. **Table 2** provides the definitions of proteinuria. The Third National Health and Nutrition Examination Survey (NHAMES III) showed that 29% of diabetics and 16% of patients with hypertension have microalbuminuria.[15]

Proteinuria has long been recognized as a potential risk factor for adverse outcomes and cardiovascular risk in particular. The Framingham investigators showed that proteinuria by dipstick was associated with adverse outcomes.[16] Microalbuminuria is an independent risk factor for CVD outcomes in multiple studies of type 1 and type 2 diabetics.[5] Albuminuria is an independent risk factor for left ventricular hypertrophy and CVD events in patients with hypertension. A population study in Norway of healthy individuals with treated hypertension but no diabetes showed an increased mortality risk associated with microalbuminuria. An ACR of 22 mg/g or greater was associated with an increased multivariate-adjusted relative risk of mortality of 7.0% in men and 6.3% in women.[17] The Losartan Intervention for End-point Reduction (LIFE) study evaluated subjects with moderately severe hypertension and electrocardiogram-documented left ventricular hypertrophy (LVH). Albuminuria was independently related to LVH[18] and increased CVD morbidity and mortality.[19] Community studies of healthy cohorts have shown a positive relationship between increasing urinary albumin concentration and mortality after adjustment for other CVD risk

Table 2
Definitions of proteinuria

Urine Collection Method	Normal	Microalbuminuria	Albuminuria or Clinical Proteinuria
Total protein			
24-hour excretion	<300 mg/d	NA	≥300 mg/d
Spot urine dipstick	<30 mg/dL	NA	≥30 mg/dL
Spot urine protein-to-creatinine ratio	<200 mg/g	NA	≥200 mg/g
Albumin			
24-hour excretion	<30 mg/d	30–300 mg/d	>300 mg/d
Spot urine albumin-specific dipstick	<3 mg/dL	>3 mg/dL	NA
Spot urine albumin-to-creatinine ratio	<17 mg/g (men) <25 mg/g (women)	17–250 mg/g (men) 24–355 mg/g (women)	>250 mg/g (men) >355 mg/g (women)

Abbreviation: NA, not applicable.
Data from Sarnak MJ, Levey AS, Schoolwerth AC, et al. Kidney disease as a risk factor for development of cardiovascular disease: a statement from the American Heart Association Councils on Kidney in Cardiovascular Disease, High Blood Pressure Research, Clinical Cardiology, and Epidemiology and Prevention. Hypertension 2003;42(5):1050–65.

factors.[20] Finally, albuminuria correlates with CVD risk in patients with known cardiovascular disease. The Heart Outcomes Prevention Evaluation (HOPE) study evaluated the risk of CVD events in high-risk individuals with a history of cardiovascular disease or diabetes and at least one other CVD risk factor. Any degree of albuminuria was found to be a risk factor for CVD events in individuals with or without diabetes.[21] The Prevention of Events with ACE Inhibition (PEACE) study assessed for the risk of death and CVD events in subjects with stable coronary disease. Albuminuria was an independent predictor of all-cause mortality and CVD events in this study population.[22]

The mechanism by which microalbuminuria may increase CVD events is unclear. Albuminuria may simply be a marker for progression of kidney disease. Progressive renal impairment may lead to worsening hypertension and dyslipidemia, as portrayed in **Fig. 1**, increasing the impact of these well-known risk factors on the cardiovascular system. Albuminuria may be a marker for the severity and duration of risk factors and therefore a marker for a higher risk population. Albuminuria may be a measure of endothelial disease in the kidney, which correlates with systemic endothelial dysfunction. Elevated urinary albumin excretion has been associated with impaired flow-mediated dilatation of the brachial artery, a measure of endothelial function, in clinically healthy subjects.[23] Finally, albuminuria may be a manifestation of chronic inflammation. In type 2 diabetes, urinary albumin excretion, endothelial dysfunction, and chronic inflammation correlate with mortality.[24] Markers of inflammation and endothelial function were found to be interrelated.

Nontraditional risk factors, including microalbuminuria, can be used to help modify a risk assessment for individual patients. The presence of one or multiple nontraditional risk factors may indicate a risk level that is higher than predicted by traditional risk factor algorithms, such as the Framingham risk calculator. More aggressive treatment targets for lipids and blood pressure may be chosen in patients that have the presence of nontraditional risk factors.

COMPLICATIONS OF DYSLIPIDEMIA IN CHRONIC KIDNEY DISEASE
Cardiovascular Disease

The increased cardiovascular risk seen in patients with CKD may be caused in part by the observed dyslipidemia commonly seen in these patients. It is common for the dyslipidemia to cluster with other common CVD risk factors, including hypertension, diabetes mellitus, inflammation, and

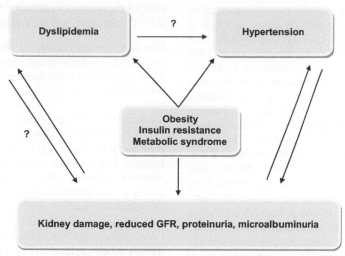

Fig. 1. Relationship between dyslipidemia, hypertension, metabolic syndrome, and kidney disease. (*Adapted from* Sahadevan M, Kasiske BL. Hyperlipidemia in kidney disease: causes and consequences. Curr Opin Nephrol Hypertens 2002;11(3):323–29; with permission).

increased oxidative stress. CVD likely develops as a consequence of the accumulation of oxidative-prone atherogenic lipoproteins, such as small, dense LDL and remnant particles and impaired HDL-mediated reverse cholesterol transport.

Progression of Renal Disease

It has long been recognized that the risk factors associated with CVD, including dyslipidemia, are also associated with the progression of renal disease. In particular, low HDL cholesterol has been associated with progression of renal disease.[25] Patients with metabolic syndrome, a clustering of obesity, hypertension, insulin resistance, and dyslipidemia, frequently have microalbuminuria, which is an early sign of renal impairment. CVD risk factors may cause vascular injury and direct kidney damage. It is also possible that kidney dysfunction can contribute to hypertension and promote other CVD risk factors, including insulin resistance and dyslipidemia leading to ongoing vascular damage (see **Fig. 1**).[26] These complications lead to a vicious cycle of ongoing endothelial damage and target organ disease and dysfunction.

Studies have suggested that the dyslipidemia of CKD may cause direct kidney damage at the glomerular and tubular level. Lipoproteins accumulate in the glomerular mesangium and may promote glomerulosclerosis. Mesangial cells take up LDL via the scavenger receptor, an unregulated process, and form foam cells.[27] Inflammatory cytokines may augment this process. Glomerular foam cells are associated with focal segmental glomerulosclerosis.[26] It is not clear if the foam cells are directly responsible for the development of glomerulosclerosis.

Reabsorption of cholesterol, fatty acids, and phospholipids by tubular epithelial cells may precipitate inflammation, foam cell formation, and tissue injury.[14] This reabsorption may be an important cause of tubulointerstitial damage in individuals with nephrotic range proteinuria.

Animal studies have provided evidence that dyslipidemia may contribute to the progression of renal disease. The obese Zucker rat, a model of metabolic syndrome, spontaneously develops progressive kidney disease. Lipid-lowering agents are able to ameliorate renal injury in this animal model suggesting that abnormal lipids may contribute to the renal dysfunction.[28] Hypercholesterolemic rabbits develop glomerular hypertrophy and injuries consistent with diffuse glomerulosclerosis. Treatment with the statin medication atorvastatin prevented most of the glomerular changes even in the presence of high cholesterol levels.[29] Finally, pharmacologic intervention to target HDL metabolism and raise HDL levels was able to slow the progression of renal disease in a rat model.[30]

Clinical studies have also suggested a link between dyslipidemia and the progression of renal disease. Early studies showed an association between obesity, proteinuria, and the development of glomerulosclerosis.[31] The Helsinki Heart Study, a primary prevention trial of middle-aged men with dyslipidemia, showed an association between renal function and dyslipidemia. Those individuals that had a higher LDL/HDL ratio had a 20% faster decline in renal function compared with individuals having a lower ratio, suggesting that blood lipids and a low HDL in particular may modify kidney function.[32] An increased serum total cholesterol level is an independent risk factor for the development of microalbuminuria in non-insulin–dependent diabetics without diabetic nephropathy.[33] A study of subjects that were newly diagnosed with type 2 diabetes who presented to the Grady Diabetes Clinic in Atlanta, Georgia identified elevated triglycerides as a risk factor for microalbuminuria.[34] This finding was recently verified in the large Atherosclerosis Risk in Communities (ARIC) study, a prospective observational cohort study of more than 15,000 white and African American participants that showed elevated triglycerides were an independent risk factor for the development of end stage renal disease over a median 16-year follow-up.[35] Although these clinical observations suggest a link between dyslipidemia and the progression of renal disease, observational studies cannot prove a cause and effect.

Treatment trials have suggested that targeting lipids may have a beneficial effect on kidney function, although results have been conflicting. An early meta-analysis of 13 prospective, small, treatment studies suggested that lipid lowering had a beneficial effect on the decline in GFR and a trend toward a reduction in proteinuria.[36] A meta-analysis evaluating the effect of statins in subjects with overt proteinuria showed that statins reduced albuminuria and that individuals with greater baseline albuminuria showed greater reductions.[37] Analysis of the Cholesterol and Recurrent Events (CARE) study, a secondary prevention post myocardial infarction trial comparing the statin pravastatin versus placebo, showed that pravastatin significantly reduced the rate of decline in renal function in individuals with more advanced renal dysfunction (GFR<40 mL/min). Subjects with proteinuria were more likely to achieve benefit from the statin.[38] A meta-analysis of subjects with chronic kidney disease and cardiovascular disease showed that statin therapy achieved a slowing of the decline in GFR and improvement in proteinuria in this subgroup.[39] The most recent and largest meta-analysis of 50 trials representing more than 30,000 subjects, however, did not show an improvement in GFR with statin therapy, although there was a significant reduction in proteinuria.[40] Overall, these studies support an anti-proteinuric effect of statins, although the effect on GFR has been variable. It is unclear if the reduction in proteinuria with statin therapy has a substantial benefit in kidney function preservation.

LIPID LOWERING THERAPY IN PATIENTS WITH CHRONIC KIDNEY DISEASE

Few randomized trials have been done in subjects with chronic kidney disease and the trials that have been completed have been small and statistically underpowered to give significant outcomes. A meta-analysis of 50 trials was performed to analyze the potential benefits of statins in subjects with chronic kidney disease.[40] Twenty-six of the trials were performed in subjects undergoing pre-dialysis. The results were mainly driven by the pravastatin pooled project (PPP) that included primary prevention subjects from the West of Scotland Coronary Prevention Study (WOSCOPS) and secondary-prevention CARE and Long-term Intervention with Pravastatin in Ischemic Disease (LIPID) study groups.[41] The meta-analysis found a significant reduction in all cause mortality (relative risk [RR] 0.81 [0.74–0.89], $P<.001$); cardiovascular mortality (RR 0.80 [0.70–0.90], $P<.001$); and cardiovascular events (RR 0.75 [0.66–0.85], $P<.001$) in subjects undergoing pre-dialysis with CKD.[40] In addition, subgroup analysis of 1329 subjects with renal impairment in the Heart Protection Study, a study comparing simvastatin 40 mg versus placebo in subjects with coronary heart disease or coronary heart equivalent disease, showed that the simvastatin was just as effective at reducing the primary end point as compared with subjects with normal renal function.[42] Post hoc analysis of the Aggressive Lipid-Lowering Initiation Abates New Cardiac Events (ALLIANCE) study investigated atorvastatin therapy versus usual care on CVD outcomes in Veterans Affairs subjects with coronary heart disease with and without CKD.[43] Atorvastatin therapy decreased CVD risk with no significant difference in treatment effect observed between subjects with and without CKD.

There is even less data available for primary prevention patients. The only completed prospective randomized clinical trial evaluating statin therapy in subjects with early CKD is the Prevention of Renal and Vascular End Stage Disease Intervention Trial (PREVENT IT) of 864 subjects with microalbuminuria randomized to pravastatin 40 mg daily or placebo.[44] The pravastatin arm achieved a non-significant 13% reduction in the primary end point of cardiovascular mortality and morbidity. This trial was statistically underpowered to prove benefit, however, because of the small number of events observed. A subgroup analysis of the primary prevention Air Force/Texas Coronary Atherosclerosis Prevention Study (AFCAPS/TexCAPS) compared lovastatin to placebo in 304 individuals with CKD without CVD and lower than average HDL. The incidence of fatal and non-fatal CVD events was lower in subjects with CKD receiving lovastatin compared with placebo and the finding was statistically significant, although the number of events was low.

The clinical data that is available suggests that statin therapy achieves a similar benefit in patients with CKD undergoing pre-dialysis as in patients with normal renal function. There is a need for larger long-term studies in this patient population to have a more definitive answer regarding CVD risk reduction in patients with CKD.

Guidelines

The National Kidney Foundation Task Force on Cardiovascular Disease in Chronic Renal Disease suggested that patients with CKD should be placed into the highest-risk category for CVD risk stratification.[3] The National Cholesterol Education Program Adult Treatment Panel III has recommended that LDL cholesterol should be the primary target of therapy for at-risk patients. Non-HDL cholesterol (total cholesterol minus HDL cholesterol) is a secondary lipid target for patients with fasting triglyceride levels greater than 200 mg/dL. **Table 3** shows the LDL and non-HDL cholesterol targets according to risk categories. Patients with CKD without documented CVD would be placed in the high-risk category. The LDL cholesterol goal is less than 100 mg/dL and the non-HDL cholesterol goal is less than 130 mg/dL. Patients with CKD and documented CVD would be placed in the very-high-risk category. The optional goal of LDL cholesterol less than 70 mg/dL and

non-HDL cholesterol less than 100 mg/dL can be considered for this category of patients.

Treatment

Prevention of CVD begins with a therapeutic lifestyle program (**Table 4**). Lifestyle changes that have been shown effective in modifying cardiovascular risk factors and reducing CVD events include reducing the intake of saturated fat and cholesterol, increasing physical activity, and weight loss. A therapeutic lifestyle diet can help reduce LDL cholesterol (**Table 5**). The Dietary Approaches to Stop Hypertension (DASH) eating plan reduces blood pressure.[45]

LDL cholesterol is the primary target of therapy to reduce CVD risk. Statins are the drug of first choice to reduce LDL cholesterol. No dose adjustments are needed for patients with mild-to-moderate renal insufficiency. For severe renal insufficiency (creatinine clearance <30 mL/min) caution is needed with some of the statins.[46] No dose adjustment is needed for atorvastatin or pravastatin. For rosuvastatin it is recommended to start with 5 mg/d and not to exceed 10 mg/d. Simvastatin should be started at 5 mg/d and lovastatin doses above 20 mg need to be used cautiously in patients with severe renal impairment. Fluvastatin doses above 40 mg/d have not been studied in severe renal insufficiency.

If statin therapy alone cannot get patients to the desired LDL goal, then combination therapy will need to be considered. Intestinal agents, such as bile acid sequestrants or ezetimibe, can be safely added to statin therapy for further LDL lowering. Colesevelam, the newest bile acid sequestrant,

---

Table 3
LDL cholesterol and non-HDL cholesterol goals according to risk categories

Risk Category	LDL Cholesterol Goal (mg/dl)	Non-HDL Cholesterol Goal (Triglycerides ≥200 mg/dL) (mg/dl)
Very high risk	<70 optional goal	<100 optional goal
High risk (CHD or CHD risk equivalent, 10-year risk >20%)	<100	<130
Moderate high risk ≥two risk factors, 10%–20% 10-year risk	<130 <100 optional goal	<160 <130 optional goal
Moderate risk ≥two risk factors, <10% 10-year risk	<130	<160
Low risk 0 or 1 risk factor	<160	<190

Data from Third Report of the National Cholesterol Education Program (NCEP) Expert Panel on Detection, Evaluation, and Treatment of High Blood Cholesterol in Adults (Adult Treatment Panel III) final report. Circulation 2002;106(25):3143–21; and Grundy SM, Cleeman JI, Merz CN, et al. Implications of recent clinical trials for the National Cholesterol Education Program Adult Treatment Panel III guidelines. Circulation 2004;110(2):227–39.

Table 4
Therapeutic lifestyle modification program to manage CVD risk factors and reduce CVD events

Weight reduction	Maintain normal body weight (BMI, 18.5–24.9)
Diet	Reduce saturated fat and cholesterol (TLC diet – see **Table 5**) For hypertension, adopt DASH diet (rich in fruits, vegetables, low-fat dairy, reduced saturated and total fat)
Dietary sodium reduction	No more than 100 mEq/d (2.4 g sodium, 6g sodium chloride)
Physical activity	Regular aerobic physical activity at least 30 min/d most days of the week
Moderate alcohol intake	Limit consumption to no more than two drinks per day in men and one drink per day in women

Abbreviations: BMI, body mass index; TLC, therapeutic lifestyle modification.

Data from Chobanian AV, Bakris GL, Black HR, et al. The seventh report of the Joint National Committee on Prevention, Detection, Evaluation, and Treatment of High Blood Pressure: the JNC 7 report. JAMA 2003;289(19):2560–72.

also improves glycemic control in patients with type 2 diabetes mellitus with a mean reduction in hemoglobin A_{1c} between 0.5% and 1% compared with placebo.[47] Outcome studies showing that combination therapy can lead to further CVD risk reduction have not been completed. The potential benefit of further LDL lowering needs to be balanced with the potential for side effects from combination therapy. In general, it is worthwhile considering more aggressive LDL lowering in the highest-risk individuals.

Non-HDL cholesterol is the secondary target of therapy after LDL lowering for individuals with fasting triglyceride levels greater than 200 mg/dL. Because most patients with CKD have a mixed hyperlipidemia with elevated triglycerides and low HDL cholesterol, non-HDL cholesterol is an important target in patients with CKD. Combination therapy will be necessary in many patients with CKD to achieve the non-HDL cholesterol goal. There are three strategies for lowering non-HDL cholesterol: further LDL cholesterol lowering, raising HDL cholesterol, or reducing triglyceride levels. It has not been determined if one strategy will lead to better outcomes over another.

There is emerging evidence that more aggressive LDL lowering may achieve greater CVD risk reductions. The Treating to New Targets (TNT) trial evaluated atorvastatin 10 mg versus atorvastatin 80 mg in subjects with chronic coronary heart disease.[48] The higher dose statin achieved a further 22% relative risk reduction (2.2% absolute risk reduction) in cardiovascular events compared with the lower dose statin with a mean LDL cholesterol of 77 mg/dL achieved in the high dose group. This study suggests that a strategy to treat the LDL cholesterol to as low a level as possible using the highest tolerable statin dose

Table 5
Nutrient composition of the therapeutic lifestyle changes diet

Saturated fat	<7% of total calories, eliminate trans fatty acids
Polyunsaturated fat	Up to 10% of total calories
Monounsaturated fat	Up to 20% of total calories
Total fat	25%–35% of total calories
Carbohydrate (from foods rich in complex carbohydrates, including whole grains, fruits, vegetables)	50%–60% of total calories
Fiber	20–30 g/d
Protein	Approximately 15% of calories
Cholesterol	<200 mg/d
Total calories	Balance energy intake and expenditure to maintain desirable body weight/prevent weight gain (include moderate physical activity)

Data from Third Report of the National Cholesterol Education Program (NCEP) Expert Panel on Detection, Evaluation, and Treatment of High Blood Cholesterol in Adults (Adult Treatment Panel III) final report. Circulation 2002;106(25):3143–21.

before considering combination therapy is a reasonable first step.

A strategy to raise HDL cholesterol can also reduce non-HDL cholesterol levels. Niacin therapy has the greatest potential to raise HDL cholesterol levels in addition to offering further LDL cholesterol lowering. There have been few outcome studies, however, that document cardiovascular risk reduction with niacin in combination with statins and limited data in patients with CKD. Tolerability may limit its use for many patients.

Reducing triglycerides will lower total cholesterol and non-HDL cholesterol. This strategy may also shift small dense LDL particles to larger, more buoyant particles. The treatment of hypertriglyceridemia consists of a combination of lifestyle modification and pharmacologic therapy when lifestyle changes alone cannot achieve the desired triglyceride goal. A diet that concentrates on reducing complex carbohydrates can lower triglyceride levels. In addition, a reduction or elimination of alcohol can be beneficial. Fish oils reduce triglycerides, although the dose needed to reduce triglycerides by about 35% are typically 3 to 4 g per day of a combination of eicosapentaenoic acid and docosahexaenoic acid.[49] Fibrates, gemfibrozil and fenofibrate, are effective agents to lower triglycerides. The National Lipid Association (NLA) Safety Task Force cautions that fibrates can increase creatinine levels, although this is usually a reversible increase that returns to baseline when the fibrate is discontinued.[50] The NLA recommends that gemfibrozil should be reduced to 600 mg/d and fenofibrate reduced to 48 mg/d for individuals with a GFR from 15 to 59 mL/min/1.73m^2. Both drugs should be avoided if the GFR is less than 15 mL/min/1.73m^2.

There are no completed studies using the combination of statins and fibrates that show an outcome advantage to this combination. There is a safety concern with this combination because of the possible increase risk for muscle toxicity and rhabdomyolysis, especially when gemfibrozil is added to a statin. The NLA recommends fenofibrate as the preferred fibrate in combination with a statin because fenofibrate uses a different hepatic enzyme that does not interfere with the metabolism of statins.[50] In addition, if a fibrate is to be used with a statin, it is advised not to use the maximal statin dose in combination.

SUMMARY

Patients with chronic kidney disease are at high cardiovascular risk and we can consider them to have a risk equivalent to coronary heart disease, putting them into the high-risk category. A mixed dyslipidemia with high triglyceride levels, low HDL levels, and small, dense LDL particles is a common pattern in patients with CKD contributing to their high CVD risk. A treatment strategy to reduce LDL cholesterol to the current high-risk category goals reduces risk similar to patients without CKD. Emerging evidence suggests that targeting non-HDL cholesterol can have the potential to bring about further CVD risk reduction. Non-HDL cholesterol should be a secondary target for all patients with CKD. Further studies are needed to determine the magnitude of the risk reduction we can expect to gain by targeting non-HDL cholesterol and the most effective way to treat this target.

REFERENCES

1. National Kidney Foundation. K/DOQI clinical practice guidelines for chronic kidney disease: evaluation, classification, and stratification. Am J Kidney Dis 2002;39(2 Suppl 1):S1–266.
2. Shulman NB, Ford CE, Hall WD, et al. Prognostic value of serum creatinine and effect of treatment of hypertension on renal function. Results from the hypertension detection and follow-up program. The Hypertension Detection and Follow-up Program Cooperative Group. Hypertension 1989;13(Suppl 5):I80–93.
3. Levey AS, Beto JA, Coronado BE, et al. Controlling the epidemic of cardiovascular disease in chronic renal disease: what do we know? What do we need to learn? Where do we go from here? National Kidney Foundation Task Force on Cardiovascular Disease. Am J Kidney Dis 1998;32(5):853–906.
4. Iseki K, Yamazato M, Tozawa M, et al. Hypocholesterolemia is a significant predictor of death in a cohort of chronic hemodialysis patients. Kidney Int 2002;61(5):1887–93.
5. Sarnak MJ, Levey AS, Schoolwerth AC, et al. Kidney disease as a risk factor for development of cardiovascular disease: a statement from the American Heart Association Councils on Kidney in Cardiovascular Disease, High Blood Pressure Research, Clinical Cardiology, and Epidemiology and Prevention. Hypertension 2003;42(5):1050–65.
6. National Cholesterol Education Program (NCEP) Expert Panel on Detection, Evaluation, and Treatment of High Blood Cholesterol in Adults (Adult Treatment Panel III). Third Report of the National Cholesterol Education Program (NCEP) Expert Panel on Detection, Evaluation, and Treatment of High Blood Cholesterol in Adults (Adult Treatment Panel III) final report. Circulation 2002;106(25):3143–421.
7. Uhlig K, Levey AS, Sarnak MJ. Traditional cardiac risk factors in individuals with chronic kidney disease. Semin Dial 2003;16(2):118–27.

8. Kasiske BL. Hyperlipidemia in patients with chronic renal disease. Am J Kidney Dis 1998;32(5 Suppl 3): S142–56.

9. Austin MA. Triglyceride, small, dense low-density lipoprotein, and the atherogenic lipoprotein phenotype. Curr Atheroscler Rep 2000;2(3):200–7.

10. Roheim PS, Asztalos BF. Clinical significance of lipoprotein size and risk for coronary atherosclerosis. Clin Chem 1995;41(1):147–52.

11. Vaziri ND, Deng G, Liang K. Hepatic HDL receptor, SR-B1 and Apo A-I expression in chronic renal failure. Nephrol Dial Transplant 1999;14(6):1462–6.

12. Vaziri ND, Moradi H. Mechanisms of dyslipidemia of chronic renal failure. Hemodial Int 2006;10(1):1–7.

13. Shearer GC, Stevenson FT, Atkinson DN, et al. Hypoalbuminemia and proteinuria contribute separately to reduced lipoprotein catabolism in the nephrotic syndrome. Kidney Int 2001;59(1):179–89.

14. Vaziri ND. Dyslipidemia of chronic renal failure: the nature, mechanisms, and potential consequences. Am J Physiol Renal Physiol 2006;290(2):F262–72.

15. Jones CA, Francis ME, Eberhardt MS, et al. Microalbuminuria in the US population: third National Health and Nutrition Examination Survey. Am J Kidney Dis 2002;39(3):445–59.

16. Kannel WB, Stampfer MJ, Castelli WP, et al. The prognostic significance of proteinuria: the Framingham study. Am Heart J 1984;108(5):1347–52.

17. Romundstad S, Holmen J, Kvenild K, et al. Microalbuminuria and all-cause mortality in 2,089 apparently healthy individuals: a 4.4-year follow-up study. The Nord-Trondelag Health Study (HUNT), Norway. Am J Kidney Dis 2003;42(3):466–73.

18. Wachtell K, Olsen MH, Dahlof B, et al. Microalbuminuria in hypertensive patients with electrocardiographic left ventricular hypertrophy: the LIFE study. J Hypertens 2002;20(3):405–12.

19. Wachtell K, Ibsen H, Olsen MH, et al. Albuminuria and cardiovascular risk in hypertensive patients with left ventricular hypertrophy: the LIFE study. Ann Intern Med 2003;139(11):901–6.

20. Hillege HL, Fidler V, Diercks GF, et al. Urinary albumin excretion predicts cardiovascular and non-cardiovascular mortality in general population. Circulation 2002;106(14):1777–82.

21. Gerstein HC, Mann JF, Yi Q, et al. Albuminuria and risk of cardiovascular events, death, and heart failure in diabetic and nondiabetic individuals. JAMA 2001;286(4):421–6.

22. Solomon SD, Lin J, Solomon CG, et al. Influence of albuminuria on cardiovascular risk in patients with stable coronary artery disease. Circulation 2007; 116(23):2687–93.

23. Clausen P, Jensen JS, Jensen G, et al. Elevated urinary albumin excretion is associated with impaired arterial dilatory capacity in clinically healthy subjects. Circulation 2001;103(14):1869–74.

24. Stehouwer CD, Gall MA, Twisk JW, et al. Increased urinary albumin excretion, endothelial dysfunction, and chronic low-grade inflammation in type 2 diabetes: progressive, interrelated, and independently associated with risk of death. Diabetes 2002;51(4): 1157–65.

25. Schaeffner ES, Kurth T, Curhan GC, et al. Cholesterol and the risk of renal dysfunction in apparently healthy men. J Am Soc Nephrol 2003; 14(8):2084–91.

26. Sahadevan M, Kasiske BL. Hyperlipidemia in kidney disease: causes and consequences. Curr Opin Nephrol Hypertens 2002;11(3):323–9.

27. Ruan XZ, Varghese Z, Powis SH, et al. Dysregulation of LDL receptor under the influence of inflammatory cytokines: a new pathway for foam cell formation. Kidney Int 2001;60(5):1716–25.

28. Kasiske BL, O'Donnell MP, Cleary MP, et al. Treatment of hyperlipidemia reduces glomerular injury in obese Zucker rats. Kidney Int 1988;33(3):667–72.

29. Vazquez-Perez S, Aragoncillo P, de Las HN, et al. Atorvastatin prevents glomerulosclerosis and renal endothelial dysfunction in hypercholesterolaemic rabbits. Nephrol Dial Transplant 2001; 16(Suppl 1):40–4.

30. Vaziri ND, Liang K. ACAT inhibition reverses LCAT deficiency and improves plasma HDL in chronic renal failure. Am J Physiol Renal Physiol 2004; 287(5):F1038–43.

31. Kasiske BL, Crosson JT. Renal disease in patients with massive obesity. Arch Intern Med 1986;146(6): 1105–9.

32. Manttari M, Tiula E, Alikoski T, et al. Effects of hypertension and dyslipidemia on the decline in renal function. Hypertension 1995;26(4):670–5.

33. Gall MA, Hougaard P, Borch-Johnsen K, et al. Risk factors for development of incipient and overt diabetic nephropathy in patients with non-insulin dependent diabetes mellitus: prospective, observational study. BMJ 1997;314(7083):783–8.

34. Kohler KA, McClellan WM, Ziemer DC, et al. Risk factors for microalbuminuria in black Americans with newly diagnosed type 2 diabetes. Am J Kidney Dis 2000;36(5):903–13.

35. Bash LD, Astor BC, Coresh J. Risk of Incident ESRD: A Comprehensive Look at Cardiovascular Risk Factors and 17 Years of Follow-up in the Atherosclerosis Risk in Communities (ARIC) Study. Am J Kidney Dis 2010;55(1):31–41.

36. Fried LF, Orchard TJ, Kasiske BL. Effect of lipid reduction on the progression of renal disease: a meta-analysis. Kidney Int 2001;59(1):260–9.

37. Douglas K, O'Malley PG, Jackson JL. Meta-analysis: the effect of statins on albuminuria. Ann Intern Med 2006;145(2):117–24.

38. Tonelli M, Moye L, Sacks FM, et al. Effect of pravastatin on loss of renal function in people with moderate

chronic renal insufficiency and cardiovascular disease. J Am Soc Nephrol 2003;14(6):1605–13.

39. Sandhu S, Wiebe N, Fried LF, et al. Statins for improving renal outcomes: a meta-analysis. J Am Soc Nephrol 2006;17(7):2006–16.

40. Strippoli GF, Navaneethan SD, Johnson DW, et al. Effects of statins in patients with chronic kidney disease: meta-analysis and meta-regression of randomised controlled trials. BMJ 2008;336(7645): 645–51.

41. Tonelli M, Isles C, Curhan GC, et al. Effect of pravastatin on cardiovascular events in people with chronic kidney disease. Circulation 2004;110(12): 1557–63.

42. Heart Protection Study Collaborative Group. MRC/BHF Heart Protection Study of cholesterol lowering with simvastatin in 20,536 high-risk individuals: a randomised placebo-controlled trial. Lancet 2002;360(9326):7–22.

43. Koren MJ, Davidson MH, Wilson DJ, et al. Focused atorvastatin therapy in managed-care patients with coronary heart disease and CKD. Am J Kidney Dis 2009;53(5):741–50.

44. Asselbergs FW, Diercks GF, Hillege HL, et al. Effects of fosinopril and pravastatin on cardiovascular events in subjects with microalbuminuria. Circulation 2004;110(18):2809–16.

45. Sacks FM, Svetkey LP, Vollmer WM, et al. Effects on blood pressure of reduced dietary sodium and the Dietary Approaches to Stop Hypertension (DASH) diet. DASH-Sodium Collaborative Research Group. N Engl J Med 2001;344(1):3–10.

46. Harper CR, Jacobson TA. Managing dyslipidemia in chronic kidney disease. J Am Coll Cardiol 2008; 51(25):2375–84.

47. Bays HE, Goldberg RB, Truitt KE, et al. Colesevelam hydrochloride therapy in patients with type 2 diabetes mellitus treated with metformin: glucose and lipid effects. Arch Intern Med 2008;168(18): 1975–83.

48. LaRosa JC, Grundy SM, Waters DD, et al. Intensive lipid lowering with atorvastatin in patients with stable coronary disease. N Engl J Med 2005;352(14): 1425–35.

49. Harris WS. n-3 fatty acids and serum lipoproteins: human studies. Am J Clin Nutr 1997;65(Suppl 5): 1645S–54S.

50. Davidson MH, Armani A, McKenney JM, et al. Safety considerations with fibrate therapy. Am J Cardiol 2007;99(6A):3C–18C.

Index

Note: Page numbers of article titles are in **boldface** type.

Moving?

Make sure your subscription moves with you!

To notify us of your new address, find your **Clinics Account Number** (located on your mailing label above your name), and contact customer service at:

Email: journalscustomerservice-usa@elsevier.com

800-654-2452 (subscribers in the U.S. & Canada)
314-447-8871 (subscribers outside of the U.S. & Canada)

Fax number: 314-447-8029

Elsevier Health Sciences Division
Subscription Customer Service
3251 Riverport Lane
Maryland Heights, MO 63043

*To ensure uninterrupted delivery of your subscription, please notify us at least 4 weeks in advance of move.

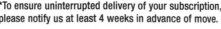

Printed and bound by CPI Group (UK) Ltd, Croydon, CR0 4YY

03/10/2024

01040354-0011